GLOBAL SCIENCE / WOMEN'S HEALTH

GLOBAL SCIENCE / WOMEN'S HEALTH

edited by
Cindy Patton and Helen Loshny

\<teneo\> // press

YOUNGSTOWN, NEW YORK

TABLE OF CONTENTS

List of Figures and Table

GLOBAL SCIENCE /
WOMEN'S HEALTH

CHAPTER 1

INTRODUCTION

Cindy Patton

The past 3 decades have witnessed unprecedented integration of global information systems. From satellite-television news to the Internet, more people share information than ever before. At the same time, biomedical research teams have increased collaborations across private and public sectors, national borders (especially by involving both the first world and third world), and disciplines. These factors have resulted in an explosion of scientific information more widely accessible than research produced a generation ago (Cameron & Stein, 2000; Castells, 2003). Gone are the days when scientists and clinicians had to wait for the publication of research results or travel to conferences to meet with peers and hunt for the latest results. Consumers of biomedical knowledge are no longer entirely at the mercy of their doctors' timetables, waiting for them to pass along new wisdom, treatments, or concepts. Consumers can access scientific results directly, and form discussion groups to assess the rapidly evolving understanding and treatment of medical conditions.

Policy makers, and the publics they are meant to represent, now exist in a strange space where lay and expert knowledge mingle, with a mind-boggling amount of information from multiple sources to sort through as they craft official and unofficial responses to public health issues (Parent, Anderson, Gleberzon, & Cutler, 2001).

While biomedical science has made tremendous strides in understanding and treating disease, the intellectual economy of global science does not draw equally on scientists from different countries. The major drug companies that support research and development of applied products of biomedical knowledge are located primarily in the United States and, to a lesser extent, Canada and the European Union. The United States has the largest number of research universities in the world, putting it in a favorable position to compete for top scientists. After the fall of communism, scientists themselves became a global commodity, either relocating to major research centers, or collaborating with those scholars and corporations best placed to support their research.

Historians and philosophers of science debate the extent to which scientific knowledge is, or can be, free of political and cultural values. However, even if we leave aside the complex questions of the dependence or independence of science(s)' epistemologies—this is a difference even among the sciences—there can be no doubt that transferring, translating, and mobilizing (not to mention withholding, obscuring, or otherwise policing the use of) knowledge is wholly imbricated in social, political, and cultural processes. This is compounded by the fact that scientists' conceptual frameworks (learned through their subdisciplines and inflected by geographically situated schools of thought) treat the idea of global disease and the possibilities of local solutions differently (Patton, 2002). The trouble with applying knowledge generated in North American or European centers—even when these "centers" are decentered via third-world collaborations, as in the case of cholera research in Bangladesh (Kamal, 2006)—has been nowhere more widely discussed than in the case of HIV. Even the early tests for HIV, piloted on North Americans, proved unusable in other contexts. This was not due to race (as in the scientific racism that underwrote the Tuskegee syphilis study or Nazi experimentation on concentration-camp internees), but to the fact that the reagents designed to react with the HIV antibody cross-reacted with antibodies endemic to people living in particular locales, especially tropical areas (and in particular, those with malaria) (Patton, 1990). Tragically, at the very moment when epidemiologists had an early chance to assess the extent of cases of HIV among women on the African subcontinent, their tests failed everyone; not only was malaria vastly more common in the region than in North America or Europe, but malaria was dramatically overrepresented in women in the region. Para-doxically, science, especially in its translation and application, can eas-ily reproduce the health disparities it purports to reduce (Shah, 2001).

There has been considerable discussion regarding the interrelation-ship between global and local forces in the context of "health," a term this volume queries, rather than taking it as a clear referent. Such work has considered the benefits and drawbacks of increasing connection and interdependency (which is not always equilateral) among people and organizations that are now connected via shared systems of knowledge, transportation, communication technologies, imagined communities, and markets. Although there is no consensus about the precise, long-term effects of globalization, or about appropriate policy responses (Ouellet, 2002), some agreement has emerged. On the one hand, potential health benefits associated with globalization include new knowledge and tech-nologies that could aid in the prevention, treatment, and surveillance of illness and disease (Labonte & Spiegel, 2001; WHO & WTO, 2002). Growth in trade may increase employment and decrease poverty, that greatest determinant of health (Dollar, 2001). On the other hand, increased individual mobility can accelerate the spread of diseases (Lee, 2001), and global employment opportunities mean health professionals can be lured to more lucrative markets, a major source of "brain drain" for many countries. Global marketing of tobacco, arms, toxic waste, and human beings (especially women) comprise what we might think of as health-damaging kinds of trade. These complex global exchanges result in both direct health-related damage, as when polluting factories move to coun-tries with fewer environmental regulations, and indirect damage, through neoliberal-inspired privatization of health, which impacts public services like water treatment and electricity (Bettcher, Yach, & Guidon, 2000; WHO & WTO, 2002). Increased economic globalization appears to result in a diminished capacity for even highly developed countries to set health policies that accord with local social and political values, including the ability to protect and promote health (Woodward, Drager, Beaglehole, et al., 2001). Democratized and democratizing countries now grapple with the pressures of participating directly (through commercial relationships) or indirectly (through debt transfers and other forms of "aid" between master and client states, even if these are mediated by transnational institutions like the World Bank and International Monetary Fund) in the world economy. Countries like Canada are experiencing an often imperceptible slide toward "market" processes for health care distribution, which diminishes the incentive to tackle root causes of illness (poverty, pollution, and poor diet). Democratizing and developing countries' health policies, especially those concerning women's reproductive freedom and the health care associated with it, are now policed by the United States, which is happy to withhold desperately needed funds until Western, right-wing, Christian concepts of marriage, family, and sexuality are adopted as "health practices"—through which abortion might be outlawed, birth control refused to the unmarried, or heterosexuality promoted in its most monogamous form (even if already proven not to be lifesaving to women).

These trends have ramifications in the arena of women's health. Changes in the economic, political, and social context result in direct and hidden changes in access to health resources, including services and health care information (Doyal, 2002; Hankivsky & Morrow, 2004; Leon, 2003). However, while transnational bodies like the UN and World Bank recognize that globalization (in the strict sense of increased transportation and economic integration) affects the health of populations, the specific effects on women are little attended to, in part because of a general privileging of the health of the work force, which is predominantly male, and in part because women are primarily conceptualized as child bearers, which necessarily circumscribes the definition of "women's health."

To date, gender-based analysis of globalization has focused mainly on the impact of structural-adjustment policies and trade agreements. The idea that the production and distribution of scientific knowledge, in itself, fails to take into account the differential distribution of women in social, cultural, and economic space, has not been taken seriously by most critics. This volume is an attempt to open a debate on this matter. We take up the question of the interrelationship between "global science" and "women's health," querying each of these four terms, while also keeping in view specific cases and spaces in which their vertiginous spin stabilizes to produce clarity about how the terms intersect.

FOUR TERMS, MANY MEANINGS

While the aim of this book is necessarily collaborative on all levels, particularly in the cumulatively constructed definitions, I take responsibility for coming up with its primary terms "under erasure," as Jacques Derrida and his early English language transposer and longtime critic, Gyatri Spivak, might describe this work. I chose "global," "science," "women," and "health," both for the productive frictions they entail, and for the blind spots they engender. I chose a forward slash ("/") between left and right groupings in the title because it seems to me that, at least at this moment, we more readily trouble global and science than we do women and health; or at least, because many of us live our intellectual and activist lives across a slash, we query global and science in our academic spaces while asserting, as if unproblematic, "*women's health.*" My hope was that by interrogating all four terms, especially in these pairings, the collaborators on this project would discover more clearly the implications of differential (or deferred) troubling, and instead would see the imbrication of the more and the less troubled terms.

"*Global*" is a word almost evacuated of meaning by the sheer volume of its current connotations. I wagered that by returning to it with fresh eyes with a group of collaborators we could pay it better notice. We might see, for example, that the production of the "global" (as has arisen as a usage in the strict neoliberal sense) implies and enables some body states to be understood as matters of "health," and others not. We might find that the troubling of the term "global" so opulently underway in the academy obscures its own assumptions about social and economic processes, and that, unearthed, these assumptions might be revealed as quaintly devoid of any engagement with poststructuralist feminist theories.

I predicted that we would feel discomfort when these meanings were paired with "*science*"—as in science bound to an economy of knowledge (or the knowledge economy) and as in a product that transcends nation, effective everywhere because presumed to be above the interests of nation. "Science," of course, is also ambiguous; it might mean systematic or disinvested, or it could mean "science as such," the particular disciplines that conceive of themselves as conducting business according to particular rules. The pairing of "science" and "health" ought also to agitate: a trick of neoliberalism's self-naturalizing strategy has been to assert that "evidence"—a term necessarily linked to "science" in our era—should provide the basis of all forms of clinical and policy practice, a neat counter to the trend prevalent since the 1980s of considering social and cultural factors as at least as important as "germs" (if not more so) in understanding health. In a single stroke, the call for "evidence-based medicine" remedicalizes vast bodily territories that had been freed from biomedicine's dominion; however much qualitative researchers want to argue for the value of their "soft sciences," they must now fight this battle on biomedicine's ground; health is once again leashed to "science."

This begs us to uncouple "women's health": charmingly, the global science/women's health project was an all-girl adventure. As feminists of widely varying types, with a lifetime of questioning women's place in society and, in particular, in the academy, we interrogated our own place in relation to the terms under erasure, including the one that was meant to refer to us. I wanted to place special emphasize on the hidden elasticity of "our" term; under global science, "woman" can mean everything from the body responsible for transmitting disease, to one who has a special role to play in saving us from harms, to she whose health is perpetually deferred—by policy, or through media representation. There is a particular concern in our individual essays to reflect on the lives of women from spaces other than our own. We have also questioned whether our research practices are capable of expanding collaborative space, especially across the power divide, in terms of setting questions and seeking their answers.

TROUBLE THE FIELD

Global Science/Women's Health is the product of several years of multiway collaboration among researchers from different disciplines and theoretical perspectives, in various stages of their research careers, with different political histories, and with different understandings of the primary terms. Nonetheless, we remain united by a conviction that the various forms of feminist thought that we represent—that we *embody*—can, and must, speak to the relationship between these terms and the intellectual and human commitments we hold dear. We understand that, to some extent, the differences in our intellectual and political perspectives are disagreements from within what is, given the enormity of the assault on women on the global scale, a rather smooth space that poststructural, liberal, and neo-Marxist feminisms have wrought. On the other hand, this sense of shared space was complicated by the reality that each of us is already engaged in battles on behalf of women in our particular domains, from within the academic and social communities in which we try to make our intellectual practice matter. In some sense (though also reluctantly), we had to withdraw from *those* worlds when we had our initial weeklong meeting for this project, in order to be free to engage one another on the questions of "global" "science"/"women's" "health."

The meeting which included several more people than ultimately contributed to this volume, was, in a word, fun. It was not easy to bridge the sometimes great distances between disciplines. Nor was it easy to navigate the minute distinctions we discovered among participants from very closely aligned theoretical frameworks. I knew everyone, but no one else knew more than two of the other participants, so there was familiarization required to acquaint ourselves with others' histories and what factors had brought us all, intellectually and politically, to a single table. The week included a mix of reading papers and discussion of the project's four terms. Great pleasure arose from not having to deal with skeptical nonfeminist colleagues who deem our modest feminisms "too political." We were also able to grapple with the "so what?" questions that are necessarily on our minds when we work within our political constituencies; there is considerable ambiguity about the value and utility of our intellectual pursuits, and it was useful, I believe, for us to understand how this tension played out for feminist scholars working across a range of political sites. We could speak with our hearts and minds among similarly situated women who experience different versions of what it is like to make intellectual and political headway in the rapidly changing context of the 21st century's waking hours. Our work, as a whole, constituted a kind of patchwork or broken mosaic of a model, and my hope in enabling this collaboration was that, across our disciplines, we could offer something very concrete to the debates on how information is generated and moved.

FROM INFORMATION FLOW TO "CONNECTIVITIES"

Because the net effect of the very divergent kinds of work in this volume is to pose a challenge to current ways of thinking about health information in a global context, I want to review some of the dominant approaches in this area, to which several pieces specifically respond, and to which others implicitly stand as disruptions. Work on health information relies on one of four approaches to explain the movement of facts and ideas from those who have generated them to those who want to use them (Landry, Amara, & Lamari, 2001).

The *science-push* model stresses the supply of advances in research findings; the researcher takes on the role of providing ideas that direct research, and there is a linear sequence from the supply of research to utilization by decision makers and practitioners. As the label suggests, in the *demand-pull* model, users become the major source of ideas for directing research (Rich, 1991). In this approach, decision makers and practitioners take on the role of customers, who utilize researchers as contractors for service. The *dissemination* model argues that a mechanism needs to be added to research activities that helps to identify useful knowledge and then transfer it to potential users. The dissemination of knowledge in this model occurs when a potential user becomes aware of research results, which necessitates that research results be accessible to potential users. Finally, the *interaction* model proposes that knowledge utilization is dependant on various disorderly interactions that occur between users and researchers, as opposed to a linear progression of researcher-to-user knowledge transfer. This last model pays greater attention to the complex relationships between researchers and users at all levels of knowledge production, dissemination, and utilization, but it fails to interrogate its own central terms: "information," "interaction," "interpretation," and so forth.

In place of these models, the essays here explore particular moments or spaces of knowledge production and knowledge movement, an approach that highlights the social embeddedness of scientists, identifies unforeseen similarities between scientific and nonscientific thinking, and de-emphasizes the separation of science and society. Each essay points to particular "hot spots" where institutions overlap or intersect with discourses in relation to local, global, national, and imagined communities. In each case, we obtain insight into the particular roles played by individual clinicians, policy makers, educators, and actors in social movements—as well as their respective institutions, professional identities, and political goals—in moving scientific ideas from domains of expertise into public domains, or, in turn, in moving social ideas and social activisms on the production of knowledge into expert domains. Several essays emphasize the role of social differences in individuals' access to and interpretation of information, while others look more closely at genres and forms as vehicles for the movement of ideas.

I struggled throughout this project, and especially as the volume was coming together, with how to articulate the commonalities and tensions among the essays. The principle problem lay in the fact that half of the essays are clearly from a poststructural framework while the other half are not. How was I to make this tension creative? How could I reveal the strengths of each form of analysis? My default approach was to construct some sort of model, which I sketched repeatedly, only to discover that I needed the dimensionality of a holograph in order to enable the reader to see the whole. Belatedly, I realized that Inderpal Grewal's (2005) notion of "connectivities" might do the job. Although she is directly speaking to the terms of feminisms, diasporas, and nationalisms, her approach to neoliberalism in *Transnational America* has broad application.

Grewal tackled the difficult task of working through a set of specific cases that reveal neoliberalism's stuck-in-place features. The examples are unique. But together, directly and indirectly, they give us a feel for neoliberalism and globalism's multiple, grounded, transmogrifying ways. Because the various fluxes and flows converge intermittently (rather than permanently) to form institutions or systems, Grewal used a series of cases to explore multilayered reproduction and disruption of the thick nodes of interconnection between elements. Splitting the difference between Marxist notions of "articulation" and Foucauldian notions of power distributed through networks (and, in my view, tipping to the latter), Grewal offered the concept of connectivies

> to suggest the degree and variety of connections that exist. The term suggests, as it does in relationship to the internet, that there are strong and weak connectivities, that it is not only the networks, as Munael Castells calls them, that we need to examine but the discourses that travel through these networks, how some get translated and transcoded, how some are unevenly connected, others strongly connected, and still others incommensurable and untranslatable. Moreover, in recalling the term "collectivities," the term "connectivities" reveals that the transnational connections here produce groups, identities, nationalism; that the power of many discourses to be understood, translated, used in a variety of sites means that subjects become constituted and connected through these new technologies and rationalities. (Grewal, 2005, p. 23)

Her subsequent discussion places the term "connectivity" under pressure, pointing out that it too means different things in different cases: access of people to systems; systems' interconnections with one another; how people are located in the world (when the term is understood metaphorically); a commodity to be sold—or rather, a "state" that information-system marketers offer for handsome prices. The term "connectivities" appealed to me as a strong concept without clear referent, a plural noun that indexed not a thing, but the actuality of a relationship that had to be investigated and described rather than assumed, cookie-cutter-like, to necessarily be present between an X and a Y. Applied in our context of global science/women's health, this seemed exactly right: that across our theoretical differences, each author had identified "connectivities" that showed the particular meanings "global science" and "women's health" had taken on in a particular nexus of power. I now want to discuss these particular connectivities, and then suggest what cross-connectivities or interconnectivities there might be between the essays in this highly interdisciplinary collection.

The first 3 chapters, drawn from medical folklore, sociology, and cultural studies, all take, as their point of departure, the interpretive process of women consumers of medical information. Chapter 2, Diane Goldstein's "Imagined Lay People and Imagined Experts: Women's Use of Health Information on the Internet," described the "technologically assisted health consumer" (p. 32) as a space or person that connects the multiple domains of medical information and misinformation with local knowledge developed in virtual support groups, to produce practices of self-diagnosis and prescription, product warning, and conspiracy-theory promulgation. Noting that several lines of research have substantially challenged the perception that patients and lay people are passive or ill-equipped to handle scientific information, Goldstein showed how the Internet-using lay public also constructs experts and frames its interpretation and use of information, in part, against these "imagined experts." Goldstein interviewed and observed women who use the Internet, and looked especially at how both lay users and conventional experts deal with the "problem" of "misinformation." Regarding warnings posted online by lay people, Goldstein saw a form of folk epidemiology struggling to gain acceptance by the imagined (but official) authorities. When these authorities return such calls to "notice disease" with warnings about "bad information," we discover that despite the apparently unconstrained connectivity of lay people and information, the existing institutions and spaces of expertise continue to have more power than these lay people.

Rachel Askew and Irene Browne took up a different dimension of consumers' use of "global information," this time in the form of direct-to-consumer advertising. Another high-water moment in the apparent liberation of information from traditional gatekeepers—doctors in particular—direct to consumer (DTC) advertisements connect consumers directly to markets, but also, to some extent, become unintended side effects of the same gendered power relations they have had the potential to disrupt. Complementing Goldstein's study, Askew and Browne reanalyzed existing U.S. national-survey work to understand women's (and especially minority women's) relationship to DTC. They found that while women actively research treatments for themselves and their family members through popular venues, the information they encounter there, while possibly improving their understanding of particular diseases and syndromes, reinvigorates the gender, class, and race stereotypes that underwrite (if not contribute to) diagnostic and therapeutic health disparities among genders, classes, and races. Relying on scientifically debunked stereotypes about which health problems are proper to which groups, DTC apparently defies the market logic of constructing consumers by "educating" individuals about potential health risks. Particularly striking is the failure of drug companies to use DTC advertisements to alert women, especially black women and poor women, to their being at higher risk for cardiovascular disease than men are. This failure results from a focus on targeting white women, which, in turn, relies on the fact that men are less likely to seek health care on their own than if a female family member takes them. Through nuanced quantitative analysis of a major survey, Askew and Browne demonstrated that despite the open distribution of information DTC enables, the advertisements themselves are "intertexts" for very conventional and problematic ideas about race, gender, and class.

Lisa Diedrich's close textual analysis of Richard Powers' historical novel *Gain* (1999), in chapter 4, may, at first glance, seem the epistemological opposite of Askew and Browne's careful quantitative analysis. Here, instead of a massive and highly representative national sample, we see one idiosyncratic novel by a scientist-turned-best-selling-novelist, and one written with highly political aims at that. However, this text also asks how information "flows"; how corporations offer and withhold knowledge; and how determinations of disease aetiology are at once intimate matters of making minute connections (in *Gain*, not only between the manufacturer of a product and cancer, but also between the development of an industry in a small town and the development of a genetic mutation in a family) and something that requires the statistical and surveillance technologies by the state (here, the Centers for Disease Control and the Environmental Protection Agency [EPA]). Diedrich reads Powers to reveal the gap between local harms and national environmental policy, but also to look at the connections that media (and to some extent, generational differences) enable; the local knowledge that too many people who live near the soap factory have succumbed to cancer is made meaningful when the daughter of an affected woman shows her a newspaper article on EPA investigations. Diedrich's reading of a novel and several ancillary texts reveals women—those with cancer, those who fear they might develop cancer, and those whose male partners have died of cancer—actively struggling to interconnect forms of information about disease: information from doctors, media, and one another. Is ovarian cancer a genetic flaw passed through generations, or mainly caused by environmental factors common to families? How many local cases are required before an "epidemic" is declared (and by whom)? Does cancer have a past (in social practices and personal habits) or a future (through genetics and poor people's inability to contest their spaces as toxic dumping groups for corporations)?

Chapter 5, the last essay in the section on connectivities from the "woman's point of view," is my own essay. It recounts my experience conducting a research project on HIV-positive persons' understandings of metabolic side effects of their medications. I discovered that the overarching failure to recognize and treat women with HIV has, ironically, led to a situation in which women are also neglected in research on and treatment of metabolic disorders. Unlike HIV, which attacks without regard to sex, these metabolic sequelae of HIV and HIV medications are highly sex differentiated, as are individuals' understandings of the meaning of them. Because HIV metabolic syndrome involves fat storage and utilization, men seem to be more subject to the cardiovascular effects. However, the causality is unclear because, as Barbara Ehrenreich (1983) noted in her eponymous book, culturally, we are more concerned about the hearts of men. The morphological changes are also confusing: in a culture in which women fear minute weight gain, "wasting" may pass less noticed than in men. To the extent that lipodystrophy also entails fat redistribution in breast tissue, women may not view this as unusual, while men see it as "growing breasts."

By analyzing gender differences in popular images of HIV before the recognition of HIV metabolic disorder, I am able to show (at least) two different interpretive communities' reworkings of medical information about HIV metabolic disorder, and to raise questions about any simple analysis that would assume "more information" is "better"; in this case, to some extent, the poor women interviewees are relieved of the burden of a suddenly transformed body image, while the gay men experience it as a crisis.

The second section comprises a cluster of contributions that track the back-and-forth movement (which is sometimes insidious) across the "/" that divides the two sets of terms underpinning this collection: "global science" on one hand, and "women's health" on the other, with special emphasis here on "global" and "women." Each essay examines real effects that occur in cases where two major and self-naturalizing themes of globalization—neoliberalism and human-rights discourse—work against the recognition of global issues as *also* being women's-health issues, and, in other cases, disingenuously take on the language of "women's health," while ignoring the real conditions of women. If the first four essays in this book highlight women's situated practices, the subsequent four essays highlight global processes and suggest that there is both value and danger, particularly with respect to women's welfare, in emphasizing "health effects" at this moment in history.

Over the past 25 years, agencies like the World Health Organization (WHO), the International Monetary Fund (IMF), and specific governments (particularly, but not exclusively, the U.S. government) have taken up the rhetoric of "women's rights" and have used the level of women's literacy, for example, as an indicator of national or regional levels of development. However, like the opportunistic feminisms of dominant political factions and governments since at least as far back as Plato's *Republic*, these moves to improve the lives of women narrow, and sometimes obviate the concerns of first world and local feminists. One vexing example is the switch in North America from liberal feminists demanding support from the state for the activities of women's groups (by funding women's centers, offering welfare packages that recognize women's particular experiences of poverty, etc.), to the state determining what will count as "women's" precisely through its neoliberal funding schemes.

As both Morrow and Hankivsky showed in different ways, issues that have been important to Western feminist efforts to end violence against women and to end women's sexual exploitation have been inexorably sutured to the neoliberal plan to devolve services to localities. For Morrow, the effort to articulate the harms of violence against women has narrowed to consider only those forms of violence that can be statistically ascribed to particular health outcomes. Where feminists once called it a social-justice issue, violence against women has since been redefined more narrowly: as a concern to the state to the extent that women's bodies have to be taken care of within the medical system. This reduction of violence against women to a "health effect of violence" has dovetailed with government funding cuts to women's group, forcing them to provide "services" identified by the government, instead of fighting the larger battle for women's autonomy and rights.

Morrow's essay explores the connections between discourses of the women's movement (sometimes deployed by activists and sometimes take up by state planners, many themselves feminists) and the specific incremental history of conceptualizing and "treating" the effects of violence.

Morrow traces the helix-like histories of the deinstitutionalization movement, feminist critiques and subsequent attempts to rework psychiatry, and the rise of neoliberalism that has rewritten the terms of all of these. She explores, in detail, the specific case of feminist attempts to cope with the shifting political climate, while sustaining a critique of the complex of systems that control women's lives as they find themselves increasingly at odds with the social movement of former psychiatric patients, who view their feminism as failing to fulfill its promise to "hear the voices of all women."

The convergence of interests between reforming feminists and the antipsychiatry movements occurs in their critique of "medicalization." However, as the governmental climate has changed toward insidiously self-naturalizing neoliberalism, the small differences in these critiques have placed the groups at tactical cross-purposes. Progressive feminists have argued, albeit not univocally, that transforming various "natural" activities or states (childbirth and menopause have been key issues) into ones that require formal medical definition and care places women's bodies in the care of misogynist systems. The antipsychiatry movement, also fraught with considerable internal differences, believes that the very concept of "mental illness" encompasses a variety of people with a dizzying array of temporary or permanent differences from a "norm" that has been identified, by default, as being the opposite of "crazy." While participants in this movement have had widely differing views on the use of physical and chemical "restraints," all agree that their voices, when heard at all, have been hijacked in the service of proving their own craziness.

The distance from "craziness" to biologically grounded psychiatric definitions is considerable when compared to, for example, HIV seropositivity. The latter is almost unarguably a "disease" with an identified cause, while it remains highly contentious whether any or all "mental illness" is importantly (or even remotely) related to biological etiologies. Thus, Morrow shows, the tension between progressive feminists and participants in the antipsychiatry movement is subjected to a strange torquing under neoliberalism: On the one hand, former psychiatric patients, to some extent, get their wish when the government sets them free from their institutions (in order to shut them down as a cost-saving measure). On the other hand, the price of this freedom is a self-normalization that has been difficult to achieve; many former psychiatric patients have been quickly transformed into criminals and miscreants and have found new homes in jails and prisons. For their part, feminists, now pressurized to articulate women's issues as women's-health issues, have tried hard to enumerate the issues faced by deinstitutionalized women, for example, a task which they have accomplished through research that demonstrates the cost to the system of dealing with these women's new health problems.

Olena Hankivsky explored the theme of global neoliberalism's appropriation of feminist ideas about human rights and shows how this results in lack of attention to the effects on women's health of the growing transnational traffic in women. For Hankivsky, the self-evidence of Ukraine's conceptualization of trafficking as a problem of morality, criminality, and human rights—a framework promoted by the United States, which, shockingly, sees itself as a leader in the fight against human trafficking (perhaps because of its spectacular innovations as a "pull" space for the trafficking in African people only a few centuries ago)—obscures the complex links between globalization, gender, and health. An explicit call to rethink even the most sedimented of policy rationales, Hankivsky described the explosion of trafficking in women in the wake of the collapse of the Soviet Union and shows how contradictory mechanisms—transnational mafias and local families, the latter hoping to help women escape their current situations—work in concert in a moment when women in postcollapse economies find themselves severely disadvantaged in new, male-oriented market economies. As global media continue to proclaim the virtues of "commodity feminism" (that is, women's right to express themselves by purchasing goods in a market economy), many women see the West as a space of freedom.

Hankivsky demonstrated that not only are the particular policies implemented by the Ukraine practically ineffective, but also that a special twist on sexism—the notion held by some Ukrainians that trafficking is understandable because Ukrainian women are the most beautiful in the world—makes it difficult to gain any consensus that trafficking in women is a problem. Hankivsky is mindful of the hazards of reframing issues in the context of a neoliberalism ready to devolve any problem to the lowest level, including the individual herself. She cautiously suggested what might be the advantages of shifting policy away from the criminality/morality framework, which runs aground on entrenched cultural assumptions about masculinity (criminal) and femininity (seductive), and from the humans-rights framework, which currently makes it all too easy for the United States to intervene (directly or through policy advice) in the affairs of other countries. Instead, she considered imagining trafficking in part, though not exclusively, as bearing a very high cost in health to women and to countries with fragile health care systems. Hankivsky argued that this approach might improve upon the human-rights framework, which has become a kind of dustbin for myriad global injustices that are structured and structure effects in radically different ways. Seeing trafficking as both a violation of human rights *and* as a hazard to health (a public good necessary for all citizens) might open up different ways for nations and transnational bodies to constitute a new social contract.

Heather Worth also considered what should be done about women's health in the context of the failure of (and failure to appropriately reconstruct) human-rights logics. In her case study of the persistent failure of global efforts to reduce the incidence and effects of HIV, Worth showed that despite overwhelming evidence about the likelihood that women tested for HIV will face many times the rate of "structural violence" of those who are not tested, or of those who test negative, WHO continues to implement HIV testing programs in low-resource countries. Acceding to an initial round of arguments about discrimination and stigma, the WHO implemented its "3 by 5" (3 million people on HIV medications by 2005) program using a "voluntary counseling and testing" (VCT) approach that assumed that people who might be infected would see treatment as a worthwhile good. This approach was destined to fail, Worth argued, because women in particular are unlikely to judge the attainment of antiretrovirals (ARVs) to be worth the violence they will probably experience after testing positive.

Global planners argue that HIV care is a human right and that, in order to provide these treatments, massive HIV-testing campaigns are necessary to identify those who could benefit. If people cannot come forward for testing voluntarily, then supporting their human rights means allowing their doctors to decide if they should be tested, an apparent reversal in policy still underwritten by rights logic. However, this also disadvantages women by failing to take into account that women are more likely to attend clinics, and therefore, that positive women are more likely than positive men to be identified. Furthermore, this use of rights logic also overlooks the now-doubled structural effects of women testing positive: as the likely first contact with the clinic, and hence testing, a woman will be the bearer of bad news to men and communities that already want to blame her for AIDS as a whole.

Worth pointed out that the malleability of human rights in the abstract persistently results in a sidelining of human rights of women in actuality; in the case of HIV, the very structural factors—feminization of poverty, the global-local persistence of sexual violence enacted on women, and the insidious disregard for women's personhood by health policy in general—that put women in harm's way for contracting HIV are the selfsame factors that inhibit the realistic implementation of HIV-treatment programs. Paradoxically, Worth noted, from a mechanical and epidemiologic perspective, it is men who are largely responsible for spreading HIV. Nonetheless, women continue to bear the burden of the social and structural effects of the illness and the pandemic. While some activists are heartened by the language and terms of the successor program to "3 by 5" ("Universal Access to HIV/AIDS Prevention, Care and Treatment"), Worth is more cautious: as long as global planning embeds a problematic understanding of women as first and foremost child-bearers and not full rights-bearing persons in their own right, then the opportunities to speak human rights in her name but not on her behalf will only multiply.

The final essay in this book works simultaneously at the highest level of abstraction and the level of personal affect. Meredith Raimondo's close reading of George Bush's 2003 tour of Africa proves Morrow, Hankivsky, and Worth's concerns about neoliberalism and its version of human rights to be well founded. The global community of journalists left few stones unturned in their exhaustive coverage of Bush's tour to, as one put it, "A Continent of Orphans" (p. 273). The images of African orphans in that coverage at once invoke their mothers—who have died of the direct and indirect effects of poverty—and leave them in the dim haze of moral ambiguity. However, since a disease—and one already visually overdetermined in the African context—is easier to think about than structural violence and the cascades of inequity that the term "poverty" means to gloss, much of the coverage uses the occasions when Bush meets people with HIV, or those they have left behind, to connect what Raimondo called "the militarization of health" (p. 273) with a particular form of affect in order to construct the first-world citizen's appropriate relationship to AIDS in the wake of the terrorist attacks of September 11, 2001 (9/11).

Raimondo demonstrated step-by-step how the Bush tour and the reportage surrounding it present these orphans as both the victims of globalization processes and terrifying specters of future terrorisms. In this move from an immediate material tragedy (Bush: "We cry for the orphan.") (p. 288) to the larger tragedy of a world held hostage by America's terrifying war (on terror), Raimondo showed how the affective relationships produced in the photojournalists' representations of the tour "construct paternalism as a necessary and appropriate response to the global pandemic" (p. 276). Indeed, the production of feeling toward the orphans serves to obscure the very people who have been failed, as is indicated by the presence of the orphans themselves: their mothers. The Bush Administration's efforts to save the orphans and to stop terrorism are really two manifestations of an impoverished and instrumentalist vision of human rights: both military and health responses are destined to do more harm to those that outgoing president has promised to help. Still, Bush cannot be called to task for either foray because the hidden figure in his picture of AIDS in Africa is a woman, whose worst crime was not having died and left her children, but rather having contracted

HIV in the first place. Raimondo suggested that any analysis that construes Bush's human-rights rhetoric as primarily dishonest underestimates the fundamental problem at the core of the very concept of human rights, and that we would be wise to understand this flaw, since we are likely to require rights as a tactic in the future. Raimondo said,

> It may be that when the President reports feeling moved, he means what he says. And it may be that some of his listeners are moved with him, in a response quite at odds with the [much cited] notion of compassion fatigue. Human rights frames engage directly in the process of subject formation through practices of identification and feeling. When coupled with discourses of citizenship that emphasize vulnerability, powerlessness, and loss, they may serve to reinforce the very global hegemonies that continue to produce and distribute different forms of illness, danger, and untimely death. (p. 304)

Raimondo admonished us to dip deep into the affective well which was built up before 9/11, but has intensified since, in order to address the "the urgent need to develop a critical stance that will serve to challenge oppressive power relations, not in a context of callous disinterest, but in one of sincere feelings for suffering Others" (p. 304).

REFERENCES

Bettcher, D., Yach, D., & Guidon, G. (2000). Global trade and health: Key linkages and future challenges. *Bulletin of the WHO, 78*(4), 521–534.

Cameron, D., & Stein, J. (2000). Globalization, culture and society: The state as a place amidst shifting spaces. *Canadian Public Policy XXVI Supplement*, S15–S34.

Castells, M. (2003). Global information capitalism. In M. McKee & A. McGrew (Eds.), *The global transformations reader: An introduction to the globalization debate* (pp. 311–334). Cambridge, UK: Polity Press in association with Blackwell.

Dollar, D. (2001). Is globalization good for your health? *Bulletin of the WHO, 79*(9), 180.

Doyal, L. (2002). Putting gender into the health and globalization debates: New perspectives and old challenges. *Third World Quarterly, 23*(3), 233–249.

Ehrenreich, B. (1983). *The hearts of men: American dreams and the flight from commitment*. New York: Anchor Books/Doubleday.

Hankivsky, O., & Morrow, M. With Aarmstrong, P., Galvin, L., and Grinvalds, H. (2004). *Trade agreements, home care and women's health*. Ottawa, Canada: Status of Women Canada.

Grewal, I. (2005). *Transnational America: Feminisms, diasporas, neoliberalisms*. Durham, NC: Duke University Press.

Kamal, S. (2006). *Local bacteria, transnational laboratory: The politics of cholera research in Bangladesh*. Unpublished master's thesis, Simon Fraser University, Vancouver, British Columbia.

Labonte, R., & Spiegel, J. (2001). *Setting global health priorities: Precis*. Discussion paper for the Institute on Population and Public Health, Toronto, Canada.

Landry, R., Amara, N., & Lamari, M. (2001). Utilization of social science research knowledge in Canada. *Research Policy, 30*, 333–349.

Lee, K. (2001). Globalization—A new agenda for health? In M. McKee, P. Garner, & R. Scott (Eds.), *International co-operation in health* (pp. 13–30). Oxford: Oxford University Press.

Leon, I. (2003). Health: A basic right or a luxury? (Human rights: Unfinished business). *Women's Health Collection Annual, 7*, 15–18.

Ouellet, R. (2002). *The effects of international trade agreements on Canadian health measures: Options for Canada with a view to the upcoming trade negotiations.* Discussion Paper 32 for the Commission on the Future of Health Care in Canada, Saskatoon, Canada.

Parent, K., Anderson, M., Gleberzon, W., & Cutler, J. (2001). *CARP's report card on home care in Canada, 2001: Home care by default not design.* Toronto, Canada: Canadian Association of Retired Persons.

Patton, C. (1990). *Inventing AIDS.* New York: Routledge.

Patton, C. (2002). *Globalizing AIDS.* Minneapolis, MN: University of Minnesota Press.

Rich, R. (1991). Knowledge creation, dissemination, and utilization. *Knowledge: The International Journal of Knowledge, 12*(3), 319–337.

Shah, N. (2001). *Contagious divides: Epidemics and race in San Francisco's Chinatown.* Berkeley, CA: University of California Press.

WHO & WTO. (2002). *WTO agreements and public health: A joint study by the WHO and WTO Secretariat.* Geneva, Switzerland: WHO/WTO.

Woodward, D., Drager, N., Beaglehole, R., & Lipson, D. (2001). *Globalization and health: A framework for analysis and action* (Paper no. WG4:10). Geneva, Switzerland: Commission on Macroeconomics and Health Working Paper Series.

CHAPTER 2

IMAGINED LAY PEOPLE AND IMAGINED EXPERTS:

WOMEN'S USE OF HEALTH INFORMATION ON THE INTERNET

Diane E. Goldstein

This chapter explores North American lay women's interaction with Web- and Internet-based health information. While access to health information on the Internet, like access to the Internet itself, is by no means equally distributed, it has made previously obscure and inaccessible medical information available for use by far greater numbers of the Internet-using lay public. Such a change in information accessibility has had a significant impact on the growing development of a new kind of medical consumerism. This has created a context for challenging the construction of health expertise; allowed the questioning of the credibility and claims of scientists, physicians, and others in positions of power; and brought to the forefront the thinking, researching, credible, political, and active lay person. As Steven Epstein (1996) noted in relation to the interventions of lay people in the evaluation of scientific claims related to HIV/AIDS, "they have made problematic our understanding of who is a 'layperson' and who is an 'expert'" (p. 3). The Web and Internet have created a new kind of medical consumer—one who has access to a proliferation of information and ideas. Researching your own syndromes and treatment on the Web, becoming knowledgeable about ever more sophisticated ways to protect yourself, communicating with others through Internet health-support groups, and passing on warnings about products, conspiracies, and misinformation, are all part of the rise of lay uses of computer technology.

The new technologically assisted health consumer is no longer forced to be a passive receptor of physicians' advice. The result is a (generally) more educated lay consumer, one who processes information and ideas from a variety of sources, including those that medical professionals might not wish to encourage or support. Conspiracy sites, hoax sites, alternative science sites, as well as natural communication in chat rooms, by e-mail, and on discussion lists, are all seen as purveyors of misinformation. Access to the Internet, proactive medical consumerism, and epidemic activism have, in the eyes of some health care agencies and health researchers, created a "lay health monster." This chapter will explore issues related to how women actually use health information on the Internet and how medical researchers perceive women as using that information.

Perceptions on the part of people in the medical field of the use of health information by members of the lay community are products of what Maranta, Guggenheim, Gisler, and Pohl (2003) referred to as the "imagined lay person":

> between expert and lay persons there is a division of labour that is based on epistemic asymmetry: the experts are supposed to be knowledgeable and the lay persons are ignorant…Within this context, 'imagined lay persons' are conceptions of lay persons as

they are manifested in the products and actions of the experts...
Imagined lay persons need not be explicit. Nor need they have
any resemblance with real lay persons. Rather imagined lay persons are functional constructs in expertise. (p. 151)

The notion of the imagined lay person is based on a deficit model, in
which the lay population is understood by experts as *tabula rasa*, ignorant of the intellectual content, research methods, and organizational
forms of science. Despite the fact that, in the real world, those who
might be considered lay persons are extremely diverse in terms of the
full range of training, competencies, and capabilities they potentially
possess (some may be trained engineers, emergency medical techni-
cians, or medical librarians), the group of imagined lay persons is taken
by experts to be an undifferentiated aggregate or collective, jointly
lacking in scientific knowledge, and constrained in both ability and
action. As Maranta et al. (2003) argued, "The experts are faced with a
structural problem in the interaction with the lay persons: they have to
integrate the lay persons' and users' standpoints without having access
to the 'real exemplars'"[1] (p. 152). The qualities of the imagined lay
person are thus functionally ascribed, indispensable abstractions that
give experts a sense of incorporating the lay community into scientific
concerns (Maranta et al., 2003, p. 155). But who is the lay community
in question here?

INTERNET MEDICAL-INFORMATION USERS IN CONTEXT

Medical or health information is consistently reported to be the most
common subject of Internet search activities in those countries with
widespread Internet use and availability. Recent studies indicate that
66% of American (Taylor, 2002) and 64% of Canadian adults (Statistics
Canada, 2004) use the Internet, and that 80% of adults who go online use
these resources to find health information (Taylor). These statistics are
echoed in other countries with high numbers of online users, including
Japan, the United Kingdom, Germany, and China. At the present time,
after the United States (with 180 million in 2003), Japan has the largest

number of online users (with 100 million in 2003). Although the United States has the largest Internet-using population, their participation level (Internet use per capita) is not the highest in the world. Internet penetration in Sweden (68%) exceeded that of the United States (60%) in 2002 (Benschop, 2005, p. 1).

The digital divide mirrors many preexisting cultural inequities. The geographically diverse nature of those countries with highest Internet usage means little when we consider that only 2% of the world population has access to the Internet, and that 88% of Internet users live in industrialized countries where only 15% of the world population resides. In Southeast Asia and Africa, less than 1% of people are online (Benschop, 2005, p. 2). Of course, the most potent factor in the determination of Internet access and use is wealth; in general, there is a clear correlation between the gross national product of a nation and the level of Internet penetration.

In North America, the digital divide falls along economic, age, ethnic, and regional fault lines, with the majority of users ensconced in the middle to upper income levels, living in urban and suburban rather than rural settings, and being white and from middle baby-boomer age groups. Have-nots include rural, isolated, and traditionally underserved populations such as those in inner-city and low-economic-status neighborhoods, and the elderly. Barriers to use naturally include cost, geographic isolation, literacy, computer skills, and institutional policies. With regard to gender, initially Internet users were largely white, male professionals, but, while statistics gathered in 1994 by Georgia Tech University found that women made up only 4% of the American online population, by 2002, they accounted for more than half of online users. (Cline & Haynes, 2001, p. 671). According to Cline and Haynes, gender difference in North American Internet use is mediated by race. While white women and men appear to have reached a 50:50 split on usage, women make up slightly more (56%) of the African American online community (p. 671).

Eighty percent of Americans who use the Internet report that they occasionally use it as a resource for finding health information (Pew,

2002). This figure decreases to 65% in Canada, but the search for health information is still reported as the third most common Canadian use of the Internet after general browsing and e-mail (Statistics Canada, 2004). The Pew Internet and American Life Project found in 2002 that women are using the Internet for gathering health-related information at a far greater rate than men (Pew, 2002). A Health on the Net Foundation survey (1999) found that 60% of respondents using the Net to locate health information were women. In general, Internet use to search for health information is greater among women with higher levels of income and education (Pandey, Hart, & Tiwary, 2003, p. 179). Interestingly, however, African American rates of using the Internet for health information are slightly higher than usage by white Americans, a statistic that complements a reported general tendency in the African American community to use the Internet for informational purposes[2] (Cline & Hayes, 2001, p. 671).

THE PROBLEM

There are more than 70,000 Web sites that disseminate health information (Cline & Hayes, 2001, p. 671). In addition to health Web pages, online health-information seekers consult online support groups; interact with health professionals by e-mail; read online medical journals and newspapers; participate in listservs or newsgroups related to health; purchase supplements, prescription drugs, and medical equipment online; and even make use of fee-based psychotherapy, by e-mail.

While women who have computer access regularly use the Internet for medical and health research, concern about the quality of that information and the ability of lay users to sift through the proliferation of claims, products, and theories has spawned something of a secondary industry. Virtually every major governmental health agency has a medical hoax Web site informing Internet users of the latest medical myths perpetuated on the Web; guides to assessing Internet health information almost outnumber the amount of information itself available through Internet searches, and numerous journals, papers, and conferences have been devoted to protecting the public from the potential harm of Internet health research.

Referred to as a "new frontier with no sheriff" and "cyber-quackery" (Ojalvo, 1996, p. 1), concerns about the use of the Internet in health decision making are expressed with passion, reinforcing conceptions of the ignorant, easily manipulated, and defenseless imagined lay person. As noted by numerous critics, health information can be posted by anyone with access to the Internet and an interest in doing so, and while there is a wealth of information available from a variety of sources, most of it is unregulated, with no guarantee of its quality available. Furthermore, commonly used search engines do not discriminate between materials provided by those with clinical expertise and those advocating for more marginal, alternative forms of healing (Hardey, 1999, p. 823). As one white paper by the Health Information Technology Institute (1999), *Criteria for Assessing the Quality of Health Information on the Internet*, noted,

> there is no field in which inaccurate, incomplete, or biased information is potentially more damaging; for example people seeking online information may be convinced to ignore their symptoms or rely on unproven treatment strategies in lieu of professional medical treatment. (p. 6)

Perhaps what most concerns those focused on quality assessment is the prevalence of medical-product advertising on the Web, and the potential for replacing medical consultation with one's own Internet-based research. Medical products drive what is considered one of the Web's most crowded marketplaces. In May of 1998, the omnipresence of medical product advertisements online resulted in a resolution by the 51st World Health Assembly requesting that the director-general of the World Health Organization develop a guide to medical products and the Internet. This was intended to serve as a model for member states to adapt, providing advice on how to obtain reliable, independent, and comparable information on medicinal products. Above all, the WHO guide encourages users to exercise caution in five areas: the use of Internet information as a replacement for consultation, verification of information sources, wariness of inflated promises, the obtainment of medical products through illegitimate channels, and avoidance of self-treatment.

In addition to the WHO guide, the American Medical Association, Health Canada, the Health on the Net Foundation, and numerous other "official sources" have released guidelines for the creation and use of medical and health information sites on the Internet (see, e.g., Health on the Net, 2005; Winker et al., 2000). These guides are all similar, focusing their concerns on issues of transparency of authorship, professionalism and legitimacy, justification of claims, currency of information, and motives of health-information sites, combined with continual warnings that the information on any Web site should support, not replace, the relationship between patient and physician.

The majority of these guides and studies perceive lay users, and particularly women, as uncritical readers who are unable to assess the credibility, authority, relevance, timeliness, or motivations of health information found on the Internet. Nevertheless, one recent U.K. survey of doctors' experiences of patients using the Internet found that 95% of the 800 clinicians surveyed reported that their patients experienced more benefits than problems from Internet health information (Potts & Wyatt, 2002). In the same breath, however, these doctors indicated that, ironically, the Internet was causing more problems for doctors. In particular, the Potts and Wyatt study found that the physicians surveyed were concerned about Internet informed patients requesting the newest or most up-to-date treatments, whether these were practically available or not. The doctors commented that patient faith in the Internet could replace faith in physicians. This sense of threat underscores the challenge to expert knowledge arising from lay access to Internet health research. "Medical dominance," noted Michael Hardey (1999),

> is challenged not only by exposing medical knowledge to the public gaze...but also by the presence of a wide range of information about and approaches to health. At the heart of medical autonomy is exclusive access to 'expert knowledge'...and the ability to define areas of expertise and practice. The Internet provides a possible threat to this situation. (pp. 822–823)

Hardey's comments clearly delineate the reaction to Internet health information by the medical community, treating it, above all else, as a means of boundary maintenance, gatekeeping, and reasserting medical dominance. He continued:

> The equity of presentation offered by the Internet dissolves the boundaries around areas of expertise upon which the professions derived much of their power. Furthermore the illusion of authority given to computer mediated material may benefit non-orthodox medicine which lacks the symbols of power and authority routinely available to orthodox medicine. This diversity and the resulting uncertain nature of Internet health information has provided grounds for dismissing the Internet as a serious tool for professionals and for others to represent it as dangerously confusing to clients. At the heart of the debate about the unity and impact of the Internet lies the question of the quality of the material that is available on it. The issue of quality can be used to illustrate how lay users define and cope with the problem and the way it is used by the medical profession to attempt to retain and redefine boundaries around medical expertise. (Hardey, 1999, p. 827)

Moreover, as Maranta et al. (2003) noted, "experts protect their status as a functional elite when they incorporate the place of the imagined lay person into their expertise" (p. 155). Part of the reordering of time and space characteristics of globalization is, as Inda and Resaldo (2002) argued, deterritorialization or "dislodging of cultural subjects and objects from particular or fixed locations in time and space," and reterritorialization or "reinsertion of culture in new time space contexts" (p. 11). While these researchers pointed out "how cultural processes readily transcend specific territorial boundaries" (Inda & Resaldo, 2002, p. 11), their use of the concept of (de)territorialization immediately brings to mind the aligned notion of territoriality, the need to defend and control one's space in the face of a threat from others.

The problem of quality that has inspired the huge number of guides and warnings is deeply rooted in a natural-science model of diagnosis and safety and effectiveness of treatment, and in the traditional role of medicine as protector of the public interest. The sites given primacy in quality guidelines and rating lists are those considered "scientific" enough, based on a privileging of materials from randomized controlled trials. Complementary approaches to treatment, even those involving well established alternatives, are discredited, while online support groups or other community or consumer based information mechanisms fall outside of the guidelines' definitions of health-information provision. The creation of quality guidelines from within the medical professions allows experts to reemphasize boundaries in ways that clearly demarcate who is inside the box of medical expertise and who is outside.

How Do Women Use Medical Information on the Internet?

Despite the proliferation of studies warning of potential harm in lay use of Internet health information, their basis remains fuzzy and leans heavily on constructions of the imagined lay person. Little exists in the way of actual qualitative studies exploring how and why women use online health information, how they assess what they find, what harm or benefits the users perceive in their search efforts, and the extent to which lay Internet research is used to complement or replace other forms of medical consultation. Clearly, lay use of health information on the Internet has created a new kind of medical consumer, one who has access to huge quantities of information. One cannot assume a priori that lay readers are simply passive receptors of the information found on the Internet. Nor can one assume that lay readers and medical researchers evaluate patients' informational needs in the same way (e.g., lay readers frequently search for autopathographies—narratives about the illness experiences of others with the same or similar condition). The means by which members of the lay community assess Internet information, and how they process that information, are both crucial to understanding vernacular health decision making. As noted previously however, "real exemplars" of lay use are not sought out, in part because face-to-face inquiry would threaten the elite status of those at the top of the one-way flow of information.

Qualitative studies that do explore how women use medical information on the Internet all indicate to some extent that lay users are conscious of issues of quality, and have developed commonsense ways of filtering material. Hardey (1999) noted that the individuals he spoke to about medical Web sites were confident in their ability to discern reliable material and adopted a reflexive approach to their searches. As one of his respondents noted,

> If you are a bit doubtful about something it is a simple matter to ask a slightly different question to get more information. I mean, one thing about the Net is that you only have to think about what you are looking for...so one piece of information makes you think a little differently so you can get a different slant on what you want. I would say that...contradictory or misleading information was not a problem any more than it is on TV or in a magazine. (Hardey, 1999, p. 828)

Those I interviewed also felt that accessing and navigating reliable sites was a matter of common sense, largely dependent on a facility with keywords and search engines, and less on medical knowledge. One said,

> You know it's all about your search words. The kids are actually far better at this then we are. It's their world. So if I can't figure out what words to use or how to get around an information problem I ask my twelve year old son. It's a computer skill—knowing the key words that will produce what you are looking for. I wanted information on migraines and food allergies and he worked it out with me. We even figured out which sites were trying to sell us supplements and we would alter our keywords to place that stuff lower in priority. (Katie M., personal communication, March 21, 2005)

Medical accuracy, legitimacy, and currency of information on Web sites were often expressed as significant concerns and were measured comparatively on the basis of consistency and repetition. One woman interviewed as part of an HRT Internet information study by Henwood, Wyatt, Hart, and Smith (2003) indicated, there are so many different sources that you can go to, so many different sites and you are able to compare them with and you find, "oh yes, it said that on the last site so that must be right." (p. 599)

One of the women I interviewed felt that health sites were so consistent, the problem was actually finding nonnormative information:

All this stuff about how hard it is to find true info on the net... Give me a break...The hard thing is to find anybody who is not towing the standard line. Jut try it—look up angina, colon cancer, you name it—it's one site after another—clones of the American Heart association—the American Cancer Association. You gotta get clever with key words to find interesting stuff. (Linda P., personal communication, March 25, 2005)

Conscious of issues pertaining to quality and concerned about bias and commercialism, a number of users specifically developed strategies to discern bias. As a vegetarian, Jane was interested in using the Web to find alternatives to dairy products as a source of calcium. She explained her search strategy:

So you go backwards actually, you find out the benefits or not the benefits of dairy produce, by looking up something that's actually opposite...I mean you could put in "dairy products" but it might not tell you what you want to know, so you think there might be another way, so I go round the back door and go to "Soya milk" and then it tells you about that. (Henwood et al., 2003, p. 600)

Some lay researchers' skepticism of commercial sources extended to concerns about "official" medical research sites and ties between medicine and the pharmaceutical industry. From Henwood and colleagues' (2003) interviews, one woman argued,

I know what the conventional thinking is which is that something in the British Medical journal or something is meant to be reliable— it's backed up by conventional research. Then the other me says "that's funded by pharmaceutical companies, they've got an axe to grind, they know what they want and there are other natural things that you can do" and so I don't consider either more reliable. I consider all of it. (Henwood, Wyatt, Hart, & Smith, p. 601)

Concerns voiced by medical researchers about the Internet replacing consultation with a physician were not borne out in interviews with women explaining how they use Web information. Most qualitative data suggests that women use the information to augment information from their physicians. A woman form Hardey's (1999) sample indicated,

> My GP is very busy and does not have time to answer questions fully. Actually it is much easier to think about what you want to ask when you look things up on the Net. I don't get that nagging feeling that I'm needlessly taking up his time. (p. 828)

Respondents to a variety of illness-specific studies on Internet use for medical information have repeatedly emphasized the use of Web sites to clarify what they feel they are not being told by doctors. One mother, commenting on her use of online information to inform herself about her son's chronic ear infections said,

> I found so much information about how these things happen, which wasn't explained to me by his doctor. I found that very informative and felt like I knew as much or more than his pediatrician on the subject...And it has been very reassuring to me to know that...If I do a little work I can be much better informed about my child's health. (Bernhardt, 2004, pp. 4–5)

A number of surveyed individuals also indicated that the availability of pictures on the Web was an important draw. One woman told me,

> I had a very strange mole that got black and blue and I was scared to death. I made an appointment with the doctor to have it checked but I was really scared. So I went onto the Mayo clinic site and there were all kinds of pictures of skin cancer. My mole didn't look like any of those. It made me feel better. My doctor said exactly the same thing. So I was happy. (Marsha M., personal communication, April 2, 2005)

All of the women I interviewed mentioned health support groups and chat rooms as the resource they appreciate the most. One said,

> My doctor has a tendency to not want to reply to questions about what's common or typical. On the support group sites you can see what other sufferers struggle with and what they do about it. You can ask a question, "I shake in the morning, does anyone else out there have that?" I learn way more that way than I ever do with my doctor. (Asia P., personal communication, April 4, 2005)

The Pew Internet and American Life Project found in their 2000 survey that more than 90% of health-information seekers search for material on physical illnesses, and roughly 47% of those seeking health information for themselves reported that their findings influenced treatment decisions (Pew, 2000). Consumers also used the Internet to obtain performance reports concerning providers, hospitals, and specialists, and to make decisions regarding employment-related health care benefits and managed care. One in four health-information seekers, according to the Pew Project, have joined an online support group (Pew, 2000).

While support groups are among the most popular health-information sites, individuals use them in a variety of ways, placing emphasis on different information features. One content analysis study of gender differences on Internet cancer-support groups found that men and women used these sites differently, with men being more than twice as likely to give information than women, and women being more than twice as likely to receive encouragement and support than men (Klemm, Hurst, Dearholt, & Trone, 1999, p. 65). The women I interviewed, however, did not indicate that they read online support groups for encouragement, but rather gave primacy to narratives of other people's experiences with an illness, and to the importance of subjective expertise. For example, one woman said,

> If you want to know about an illness of course you should go to someone who has it. I know they might not have your form of it or their body might respond differently but that's why there is so much discussion on support group lists. I want to hear about what they

had happen to them, what they find helps. Let's face it—the docs only have certain information. You need to go to the sick people for real info. (Frankie B., personal communication, March 1, 2005)

While autopathologies (or narratives of illness experiences) were important to most of the support-group readers to whom I spoke, several mentioned the unique expertise of online members. As one woman said, "they make it their job to know all there is to know about their illness, and they tend to be open to new possibilities for research, treatment and lifestyle" (Asia P., personal communication, April 4, 2005). Working with a group of menopause support-group members (Goldstein, 2000), I found that individuals who were new or occasional list readers often wrote in to the list to explore symptoms they found to be disturbing but that did not fit standard biomedical descriptions. Bad dreams, loss of creativity, rage, and other symptoms were disturbing to sufferers but fell well outside of their physicians' frame of reference. Support groups and consumer- or community-based Web sites frequently highlight differences in biomedical and lay understandings of what constitutes necessary information concerning a condition, diagnosis, treatment, and support. Vernacular concerns about symptoms and treatment expectations were often matched more closely in support-group discussions than in online physician-based reference pages.

The survey and interview information on how women actually use health information on the Internet suggests that they are indeed critical readers, conscious of Web-site motivations, commercialization, timeliness, authority, and legitimacy, and that they employ or know of strategies to combat spurious information and bias. Seen in this light, the myriad guides exerting quality control over Internet medical information appear to be primarily territorial, a reaction to the rise of lay expertise and the questioning of medical authority, and an attempt to assert a "gold standard" for appropriate expertise and information while discrediting all health knowledge save what falls within their own narrowly defined parameters. Interestingly, quality control guidelines themselves do not always live up to the standards they assert. Transparency of motive or bias, for example, is rarely present in these guides.

As Hardey (1999) noted, a survey of 47 instruments used to indicate quality on such sites revealed that only 14 made explicit the criteria used in ranking. A 2004 study of inaccurate information about Lyme disease on the Internet determined that all sites containing anecdotal stories or personal accounts and all sites not written in English should remain outside of the survey, suggesting that such sites were unlikely to affect patient choices (Cooper & Feder, 2004). Clearly, the lay importance of autopathographies suggests that the very sites excluded from study are those most likely to actually be read by patients.

THE BAD STUFF: DISINFORMATION AND MEDICAL RUMOR

While Web-site use and participation in online support groups and chat rooms are two kinds of interactions with health information on the Internet, another situation that also concerns medical researchers and health care agencies, and one which becomes the metaphor for all that is naive about the imagined lay person, is the perpetuation of health rumors, hoaxes, and disinformation transmitted through personal e-mail warnings and news-list postings, or displayed on popular Web sites. Health-product warnings are particularly popular among women and spread like wildfire. Recent e-mail product warnings have included the following: that the artificial sweetener aspartame is responsible for an epidemic of multiple sclerosis and systemic lupus; that Proctor and Gamble pot scrubber sponges contain a dangerous derivative of Agent Orange; that shampoos containing sodium laureth sulfate cause cancer; that tampon manufacturers are using asbestos in their products to promote bleeding; that antiperspirants cause breast cancer; that the popular drink Mountain Dew will shrink testicles and lower sperm count; and that bananas imported from Costa Rica are infected with necrotizing fascitis, or flesh-eating disease.

The postings typically take the form of a warning notice, followed by a personal experience narrative, followed by an explanation of the toxin, and signed (generally) by a health care worker, official from a police department or the Centers For Disease Control (CDC), or someone else "official" sounding. Most of us are all too familiar with these warnings, which tend to come in multiple copies and crowd our e-mail inboxes. I quote here a posting I received on November 19, 2000. Within the space of an hour I received this message four times, all instances having been forwarded as mass postings to university women's discussion lists and academic organization lists. The e-mail warned,

> Please read this...very important. Some time ago, I attended a breast cancer awareness seminar put on by Terry Berk with support from Dan Sullivan. During the Q and A period, I asked why the most common area for Breast Cancer was near the armpit. My question could not be answered at that time. This e-mail was just sent to me and I found it interesting that my question has been answered. I challenge you all to rethink your everyday use of a product that could ultimately lead to terminal illness. As of today I will change my use.
>
> A friend forwarded this to me. I showed it to a friend going through chemotherapy and she said she learned this fact in a support group recently. I wish i had known it 14 years ago. I just got information from a health seminar that I would like to share.
>
> The leading cause of breast cancer is the use of antiperspirant. What? A concentration of toxins. And leads to cell mutations: AkA cancer. Yes. Antiperspirant. Most of the products out there are an antiperspirant/deodorant combination—so go home and check. Deodorant is fine, antiperspirant is not. Here's why. The human body has a few areas that it uses to purge toxins; behind the knees, behind the ears, groin area and armpits. The toxins are purged in the form of perspiration. Antiperspirant, as the name clearly indicates, prevents you from perspiring, thereby inhibiting the body from purging toxins from below the armpits. These toxins do not magically disappear. Instead the body deposits them in the lymph nodes below the arms since it cannot sweat them out. Nearly all of breast cancer tumours occur in the upper outside quadrant of the breast area. This is precisely where the lymph nodes are located. Additionally, men are less likely (but not completely exempt) to develop breast cancer prompted by antiperspirant usage because most of the antiperspirant product is caught in

their hair and is not directly applied to the skin. Women who apply antiperspirant right after shaving increase the risk further because shaving causes almost imperceptible nicks in the skin which give chemicals entrance into the body from the armpit area. Please pass this along to anyone you care about. Breast cancer is becoming frighteningly common. This awareness may save lives. If you are sceptical about these findings, I urge you to do some research for yourself. You will arrive at the same conclusions, I assure you. PS Buy deodorant without aluminium - Innoxia and Avon both have good inexpensive ones, also health shops. Antiperspirant has been linked to Alzheimers and chronic fatigue syndrome because of the aluminium content. The e-mail was signed, Katrina Scott, Assistant Director of Sports Marketing, University of Maryland. (Anonymous e-mail, received November 19, 2000)

As a result of the popularity of these warnings, Health Canada and the Centers for Disease Control, as well as numerous other governmental agencies, have created medical rumor and hoax Web sites dedicated to dispelling popular information which they see as inaccurate or risky. The United States Information Agency (USIA) also employs a Program Officer for Countering Misinformation and Disinformation, charged with responding to false stories considered to pose a risk to the United States and its citizens, many of which are health related (Castaneda, 2000, p. 137).

Although product health warnings are frequently evoked as a perfect example of the dangers of the Internet in terms of spurious health information, the warnings are instructive as vernacular statements. Whether true or false, product health warnings are framed as a form of social activism, as a posting by a lay health consumer empowered by a sense of new access to health research and a fast means to spread the word. One writer on a discussion list angrily referred to these warnings as slacker activism or slactivism, which he defined as "the art of hitting forward on your e-mail and mindlessly sending forth semi-information relating to any number of dubious causes propagated on the Internet, usernet, or via e-mail as a means of social activism" (alt.folklore.urban discussion list, 2002).

No matter how easy transmission of the message is, the messages themselves are cultural critiques, generally implicating government, big business, and medicine. Not unlike the construction of the imagined lay person in Internet-quality discourses, the e-mailed women's-health warnings construct an imagined expert—greedy, involved in conspiracy, and suppressing dangerous information. In the United States and Canada, the majority of warnings assert that the product manufacturers conspire with the Food and Drug Administration, the Centers for Disease Control, or top government officials, in order to suppress damaging information about the medical dangers of a product. The aspartame warning, for example, argues,

> There were Congressional hearings when aspartame was included in 100 different products. Since this initial hearing there have been two hearings but to no avail. Nothing has been done. The drug and chemical lobbies have very deep pockets. But there are over 5000 products containing this chemical. (Urban Legend Reference Pages, 2005b)

Most of these warnings point the finger at conspiracies, with the motives of medicine and big business characterized as capitalistic greed. The company knows the dangers, but continues to adulterate the product to maintain profits. The shampoo warning noted,

> so I called one company and I told them their product contained a substance that will cause people to have cancer. They said, yeah, we know about it but there is nothing we can do because we need that substance to create foam. (Urban Legend Reference Pages, 2005c)

Many of the Internet warnings implicitly condemn women for placing priority on their appearance or the trivial functions of purchased products. Many then go on to reject such characterizations. The tampon warning is a good example of this.

> We need to make our voices heard. Tell people. Everyone. Inform them. We are being manipulated by this industry and the government, let's do something about it. Let them know that we demand a safe product—all cotton unbleached tampons. Change to this safer tampon and give the government the word that we won't let

our monthly cycles be used against us. (Urban Legend Reference Pages, 2005a)

In many ways then, Internet health warnings are consistent with the folk epidemiological process; that is, the process by which lay persons gather observational data and other information and then marshal the knowledge and resources of others in the community to investigate unknown factors in the transmission of disease (Brown, 1992). The process generally begins with the observation of a trend of a particular illness or set of symptoms within the community, followed by a hypothesis of a connection between health effects and local pollutants. Then community members share the information and begin to consult research, ultimately demanding government intervention.

It would be easy to dismiss Internet product warnings as simply being hoaxes or "medical myths," but to do so is to deny their popular appeal, their cultural critique, and their perception of the imagined expert. I asked one woman who sent me a warning recently why she was forwarding it. She replied,

> I believe this information is covered up. They don't do the tests to really find out about the product and then when they do—woops it's too late. And by then, well we're makin' lots of money so we can't disturb the market. True or not true—we all know THAT'S true and there's no harm in keeping everyone sensitive to that. (Tanya S., personal communication, April 2, 2005)

While Internet quality guides focus on imagined lay women as uncritical readers unable to assess the credibility, authority, relevance, timeliness, or motivations of health information found on the Internet, women assert that the Internet provides consumers with an opportunity to make up for negative motivations and a lack of credibility, authority, relevance, and timeliness on the part of medicine, health care bodies, and government. The imagined expert mirrors the imagined lay person.

Concerns about patients knowing too much reflect the philosophical premise that the public should submit uncritically to the claims of experts who know better and who can act on behalf of the common good. These experts, such as the writers of quality guidelines, preserve their authority through claims of dispassionate objectivity, which allows them to weigh information and make decisions without psychological, social, or cultural issues clouding their judgment. Patients and health consumers are seen in this formulation as too subjective, too "in the moment," and too self-interested to process health information and address larger medical needs. Within this framework, situated or vernacular knowledges are seen as unacceptable, trivial, chaotic, misleading, and fragmented. In this essentially positivist construction of imagined lay people and imagined experts, all information and all knowledges concerning health require mediation by experts. The lay use of the Internet and its associated support groups, chat mechanisms, and health warnings demonstrate vernacular responses to both the rise of the educated lay person and the bloating of medical authority.

References

Allen, J., & Hamnett, C. (1995). Introduction. In Allen, J., & Hamnett, C. (Eds.), *A shrinking world? Global unevenness and inequality* (pp. 1–10). New York: Oxford University Press.

Alt.folk.urban discussion list. (2002). Posting dated January 18.

Benschop, A. (2005). *Peculiarities of cyberspace, Internet use(rs): Demography and geography of the Internet* (Report). Commissioned and published by The Sociosite Project. Retrieved March 10, 2005, from http://www2.fmg.uva.nl/sociosite/websoc/demography.html

Bernhardt, J., & Felter, E. (2004). Online pediatric information seeking among mothers of young children: Results from a qualitative study using focus groups. *Journal of Medical Internet Research, 6*(1), E7.

Brown, P. (1992). Popular epidemiology and toxic waste contamination: Lay and professional ways of knowing. *Journal of Health and Social Behavior, 33*(3), 267–281.

Castaneda, C. (2000). Child organ-stealing stories: Risk, rumour and reproductive strategies. In Adam, B. & van Loon, J. (Eds.), *The risk society and beyond: Critical issues for social theory* (pp. 137–153). London: Sage Publications.

Cooper, J., & Feder, H., Jr. (2004). Inaccurate information about Lyme disease on the Internet. *Pediatric Infectious Disease Journal, 23*(12), 1105–1108.

Cline, R., & Haynes, K. (2001). Consumer health information seeking on the Internet: The state of the art. *Health Education Research 16*(6), 671–692.

Epstein, S. (1996). *Impure Science: AIDS activism and the politics of knowledge.* Berkeley, CA: University of California Press.

Goldstein, D. (2000). "When ovaries retire": Contrasting women's experiences with feminist and medical models of menopause. *Health 4*(3), 309–323.

Health on the Net Foundation (1999). *HON's fourth survey on the use of the Internet for medical and health purposes.* Retrieved April 10, 2005, from http://www.hon.ch/Survey/ResumeApr99.html

Health on the Net Foundation. (2005). *HON code of conduct (HONcode) for medical and health Web sites.* Retrieved April 10, 2005, from http://www.hon.ch/Conduct.html

Health Information Technology Institute. (1999). *White paper: Criteria for assessing the quality of health information on the Internet.* Retrieved March 4, 2005, from http://hitiweb.mitretek.org/docs/criteria.html

Henwood, F., Wyatt, S., Hart, A., & Smith, J. (2003). "Ignorance is bliss sometimes": Constraints on the emergence of the "informed patient" in the changing landscapes of health information. *Sociology of Health and Illness, 25*(6), 589–607.

Hardey, M. (1999). Doctor in the house: The Internet as a source of lay health knowledge and the challenge to expertise. *Sociology of Health and Illness, 21*(6), 820–835.

Inda, J., & Rosaldo, R. (2002). *The Anthropology of globalization: A reader.* Oxford: Blackwell.

Klemm, P., Hurst, M., Dearholt, S., & Trone, S. (1999). Cyber solace–Gender differences on Internet cancer support groups. *Computers in Nursing 17*(2), 65–72.

Maranta, A., Guggenheim, M., Gisler, P., & Pohl, C. (2003). The reality of experts and the imagined lay person. *Acta Sociologica, 46*(2), 150–165.

Nicholson, W., Grason, H., & Powe, N. (2003). The relationship of race to women's use of health information resources. *American Journal of Obstetrics & Gynecology, 188*, 580–585.

Ojalvo, H. (1996, December). Online advice: good medicine or cyber-quackery? *American College of Physicians Observer*, 1–4.

Pandey, S., Hart, J., & Tiwary, S. (2003). Women's health and the Internet: Understanding emerging trends and implications. *Social Science & Medicine, 56*(1), 179–191.

Pew Internet & American Life Project. (1999). *Who is not online?* Retrieved April 10, 2005, from http://www.pewinternet.org/PPF/c/5/topics.asp

Pew Internet & American Life Project. (2000). *The online health care revolution.* Retrieved April 10, 2005, from http://www.pewinternet.org/PPF/c/5/topics.asp

Pew Internet & American Life Project. (2001). *Testimony to the White House Commission on complementary and alternative medicine policy.* Retrieved April 10, 2005, from http://www.pewinternet.org/PPF/c/5/topics.asp

Pew Internet & American Life Project. (2002). *Vital decisions.* Retrieved April 10, 2005, from http://www.pewinternet.org/PPF/c/5/topics.asp

Potts, H., & Wyatt, J. (2002). Survey of doctors' experience of patients using the Internet. *Journal of Medical Internet Research, 4*(1), E5.

Statistics Canada. (2004). *Household Internet survey.* Retrieved July 8, 2005, from http://www.statcan.ca/Daily/English/040708/d040708a.htm

Taylor, H. (2002). *Internet penetration at 66% of adults (137 million) nationwide.* Harris Poll 18, Published by Harris Interactive. Retrieved April 17, 2005, from http://www.harrisinteractive.com/harris_poll/index.asp?PID=295

Urban legend reference pages. (2005a). *Asbestos in tampons.* Retrieved April 2005 from http://www.snopes.com/medical/toxins/tampon.asp

Urban legend reference pages. (2005b.) *Kiss my aspartame.* Retrieved April 2005 from http://www.snopes.com/medical/toxins/aspartame.asp

Urban legend reference pages. (2005c). *Shampoo scam.* Retrieved April 2005 from http://www.snopes.com/inboxer/household/shampoo.asp

Winker, A., Flanagin, A. Chi-Lum, B., White, J., Andrews, K., Kennett, R., et al. (2000). Guidelines for medical and health information sites on the Internet: Principles governing AMA Web sites. *Journal of the American Medical Association, 283*(12), 1600–1606.

World Health Organization (WHO). (1999). *Medical products and the Internet* (Publication of the Department of Essential Drugs and Other Medicines, Quality Schools Model 99. 4). Retrieved April 10, 2005, from http://www.tga.gov.au/docs/html/whointer.htm

ENDNOTES

1. By real exemplars, Maranta et al. (2003) referred to the lack of direct face-to-face contact with lay persons as principals. The interaction becomes dependent on the way lay people are conceptualized by scientists.
2. Findings based on race are mixed. The statistic noted here seriously diverges from results by Nicholson, Grason, and Powe (2003) who, in a 1999 sample study of 509 women, found a much larger racial disparity in women's use of health-information resources; they suggested that the black women in the study had a 70% lower likelihood of using computers as sources of health information than white women did (p. 583).

CHAPTER 3

DIRECT-TO-CONSUMER ADVERTISING AND WOMEN'S HEALTH:

EDUCATING PATIENTS OR REINFORCING GENDER-, RACE-, AND CLASS-BASED DISPARITIES IN U.S. HEALTH CARE?

Rachel Askew and Irene Browne

INTRODUCTION

Due to recent changes in drug regulation, direct-to-consumer advertising—the advertising of prescription drugs directly to consumers through the lay media—has become nearly ubiquitous within the United States. Direct-to-consumer advertising (DTCA) carries the potential both to educate patients and to mislead them, and recent research has sought to identify DTCA's effects on consumers, as well as to gauge consumers' attitudes toward such advertisements. To date, this research has focused on general trends without examining the differential health impacts that direct-to-consumer (DTC) advertisements may have on specific subgroups of Americans. In particular, it would be valuable to consider gender, given that men and women differ markedly in the ways that they perceive and evaluate their health needs (Courtenay, McCreary, & Merighi, 2002; Stanton & Courtenay, 2004; Stewart, Abbey, Shnek, Irvine, & Grace, 2004; Waldron, 1997), and the ways that they seek medical treatment (Green & Pope, 1999) and experience it (Munch, 2004; Laurence & Weinhouse, 1997; Raine, 2000; Roter & Hall, 1997). Because both patients and physicians view health through gendered lenses, DTCA carries the potential to affect women and men differently.

Analyzing data from a nationally representative survey of the U.S. population, this chapter contributes to research on DTCA by examining whether women and men (1) are equally likely to be exposed to DTCA, (2) are differentially motivated to consult with their health care providers about DTCA, and (3) receive different types of interventions and diagnoses as a result of DTCA-induced physician visits. Given that health outcomes and attitudes in the United States are differentially distributed by race and class (Williams & Collins, 1999) as well as by gender, this chapter also explores race and class differences among women, in relation to their responses to DTCA and their experiences with DTCA-induced physician visits.

We begin the chapter by providing some background on DTC advertisements in the United States, outlining arguments voiced by both supporters and opponents of DTCA. We next outline extant empirical research on the effects of DTCA and identify areas where gaps in the literature remain. From there, we highlight certain gender-based disparities in American medicine and detail DTC advertisements' potential for narrowing such disparities. Finally, we present our analyses of a recent, nationally representative survey of U.S. consumers. These analyses suggest that although DTCA may have the potential to narrow disparities in

U.S. health care through patient education, in reality, direct-to-consumer advertisements of prescription drugs serve to reinforce existing diagnostic and therapeutic disparities in care.

BACKGROUND ON DIRECT-TO-CONSUMER ADVERTISEMENTS

Direct-to-consumer advertising bypasses physicians and goes straight to the consumer via mass media such as television, magazines, radio, and the Internet. Prescription advertisements directed at consumers are currently among the most common forms of health communication reaching the American public (Brownfield, Bernhardt, Phan, Williams, & Parker, 2004). This is significant since, for most of the 20th century, pharmaceutical companies advertised prescription drugs primarily to physicians by placing advertisements in medical journals. Beginning in the 1980s, pharmaceutical companies began marketing prescription drugs directly to consumers (Lyles, 2002). These advertisements tended to be in print form (rather than broadcast) due to the Food and Drug Administration (FDA) requirement that a DTC advertisement include a brief summary of indications, side effects, and contraindications that, despite its name, was often anything but brief. In 1997, however, the FDA relaxed that requirement, leading to an upsurge in the number of DTC advertisements appearing on television. The new FDA requirements only mandate that an advertisement present a "fair and balanced" picture of risks and benefits to the consumer, as long as it directs consumers to other sources of information about the drug and/or the condition it is intended to treat. The preponderance of DTCA has had a global impact, for while it is currently only allowed in the United States and New Zealand, many nations inadvertently receive a plentiful dose of the advertisements through imported U.S. newspapers, magazines, and cable feed.

The FDA's relaxation of DTCA guidelines led to enormous spending increases on DTC advertising by pharmaceutical companies. From 1997 to 2001 budgets for DTCA increased by 145%, compared to the 66% increase seen in other promotional spending (Gahart, Duhamel,

Dievler, & Price, 2003). Spending on DTCA has continued to rise, according to industry estimates, to \$3.2 billion in 2003, and to more than \$4.2 billion in 2005 (IMS Health, 2006).

In response to this growing trend, two divergent camps have emerged to voice their opinions on the likely impact that DTCA will have on the American public. The pro-DTCA camp views these advertisements as offering consumers important health information about treatments and undiagnosed conditions, either directly, through the advertisements themselves, or indirectly, by pointing consumers to external sources of health information. For example, Alan Holmer, former president of the Pharmaceutical Research and Manufacturers of America, pointed to the widespread extent of undiagnosed chronic illnesses like cardiovascular disease (CVD) and depression, and suggested DTC advertisements will help the American public recognize risk factors of such ailments and consequently contact their health care providers (Holmer, 1999). Proponents of DTCA also said the advertisements empower patients to take a more active role in their own health care (Perri, Shinde, & Banavali, 1999), improve adherence to prescribed drug regimens, and facilitate doctor-patient communication (Holmer 1999, 2002; Krieger, 1998). Moreover, they argued, advertising directly to the public is ultimately safe, since physicians must still decide whether or not to prescribe a drug (Calfee, 2002).

The anti-DTCA camp opposes DTCA on the grounds that the objectives of drug promotion and health education are inherently at odds. These advertisements mislead, they say, by highlighting a drug's benefits and playing down its risks. As one set of critics put it, "Such advertising does increase awareness of drugs, but its purpose, as with all advertising, is to persuade rather than to inform" (Mansfield, Mintzes, Richards, & Toop, 2005, p. 6). Opponents of DTCA are also concerned with how little authority the FDA has to discipline pharmaceutical companies whose advertisements disseminate misleading information about their products or are otherwise in violation of current FDA regulations (Gahart et al., 2003). Others point out that these advertisements tend to promote the newest, most expensive treatments, rather than the most appropriate ones (Mansfield & Mintzes, 2003); that they promote the medicalization of natural processes like menopause (Conrad & Leiter, 2004); and that DTCA will drive up the cost of health care in general, and prescription drugs in particular, both because the advertisements stimulate demand for drugs, and because pharmaceutical companies pass the cost of advertisements on to consumers (Vogel, Ramachandran, & Zachry, 2003). Finally, critics of DTCA suggest that it erodes the doctor-patient relationship by challenging physician autonomy and promoting doctor shopping in the case of a physician who refuses to prescribe a desired drug (Bell, Wilkes, & Kravitz, 1999). As a result, say its opponents, DTCA leads doctors to prescribe unwarranted drugs in a bid not to alienate patients or to lose their business altogether (Mintzes et al., 2003).

EXISTING RESEARCH ON DIRECT-TO-CONSUMER ADVERTISEMENTS

Research on direct-to-consumer advertisements suggests that the explosion of DTCA in the years following 1997 unsurprisingly led to increased visibility of these advertisements. For example, an FDA patient survey found that 72% of American adults had seen or heard a direct-to-consumer advertisement in 1999. By 2002, the percentage had risen to 81% (Aikin, Swasy, & Braman, 2004). Similarly, a recent telephone survey of the American public, conducted between March, 2000, and March, 2001, indicated that 83% of Americans had seen or heard a DTC advertisement in the previous 12 months (Murray et al. 2004).

In addition to becoming more aware of direct-to-consumer advertisements, American consumers are also reporting a generally positive reaction to them. A recent survey on public perceptions of DTCA found that the vast majority (88%) believe advertisements give patients confidence to talk to their doctors about their concerns; 72% also believe the advertisements improve people's understanding of medical conditions and treatments (Murray et al., 2004). Nevertheless, the same survey found consumers are also wary of the advertisements' potentially deleterious effects. The majority (76%) believe advertisements drive up the cost of prescription drugs, and nearly half (48%) believe advertisements promote unnecessary visits (Murray, Lo, Pollack, Donelan, & Lee, 2004). It is worth noting that some consumers' optimism towards DTC advertisements may be due to their overestimation of the FDA's level of regulation. For example, a recent survey of adults in Sacramento, CA, found that 42% of respondents believed only "completely safe" drugs could be advertised directly to the public (Bell, Kravitz, & Wilkes, 1999).

DTCA does appear to affect physicians' prescribing practices. A 2002 report by the U.S. General Accounting Office (2002) reported that each 10% increase in DTCA spending within a drug class increases sales in that class by 1%. Moreover, a set of surveys conducted by Prevention Magazine (2001) found that 71% of patients who ask for an advertised drug receive that drug. Additionally, a randomized, controlled trial of the effect of patients' requests for a DTC-advertised antidepressant drug on physician prescribing found that patients who requested a DTC-advertised drug were significantly more likely to obtain a prescription than were those patients who presented with the same symptoms but made no such request (Kravitz et al., 2005).

Finally, preliminary evidence suggests that the general educational value of DTCA may be oversold by proponents. Rather than providing consumers with information on a wide variety of drugs and medical conditions, these promotions inform consumers about a smaller subset of available prescription drugs. In 2000, 60% of industry spending on DTCA went into promoting just 20 prescription drugs (Rosenthal, Berndt, Donohue, Frank, & Epstein, 2002). Furthermore, while consumers may remember the names of particular drugs, they are much less likely to remember information about the purpose of the drug, its efficacy level, and its side effects.

WHY STUDY DIRECT-TO-CONSUMER ADVERTISING'S EFFECTS ON SUBGROUPS OF AMERICANS?

To date, to our knowledge, empirical research on DTCA has focused almost exclusively on the American population as a whole rather than on the differential impact DTC advertisements may have on subgroups of Americans. This broad focus may mask significant differences in exposure to and impact of DTC advertisements. DTC advertisements are a public good, educating consumers about their health care choices, or an unnecessary evil, misleading patients or consumers and driving up health care costs, two pertinent questions remain: Which demographic groups are more likely to see such advertisements? Whether one believes DTC advertisements are a public good that educates consumers about health care choices, or an unnecessary evil that misleads consumers and drives up health care costs, two pertinent questions remain: Which demographic groups are more likely to see such advertisements? Which demographic groups are more likely to respond to DTCA?

In *Breaking Up America: Advertisers and the New Media World* (1997), Joseph Turow described how advertisers in the late 20th and early 21st century are increasingly moving away from mass-marketing campaigns that involve promoting a product to people irrespective of their lifestyles and backgrounds, and moving toward intentional targeting of particular groups and even individuals based on their race, gender, age, zip code, or other defining characteristics. Targeting activities include marketing particular products to certain groups and not to others, as well as marketing the same product to different demographic groups using different promotional techniques. Turow (1997) demonstrated that advertisers in the 21st century are increasingly working with media firms to "separate audiences into different worlds according to distinctions that ad people feel make the audiences feel secure and comfortable" (Turow, 1997, p. 2). Advertisers seek to exploit and promote existing differences between groups in an effort to create "primary media communities" (Turow, 1997, p. 4) that are formed when consumers feel that a TV channel or magazine resonates with them, reaches people like them, and excludes people who do not share their values, beliefs, or lifestyle. Advertisers able to cultivate and subsequently tap into these primary media communities can efficiently target these specific audiences with their advertisements. While targeting may be a successful advertising technique, increasing the likelihood that those viewing or hearing advertisements for certain products are those most likely to buy those products, it also leads to an uneven distribution of information about available products and services making its way to different groups of consumers.

Even among those groups targeted by DTC advertisements, however, exposure to DTC advertisements does not necessarily equate with being better informed about one's health care options. For example, older people, with their higher utilization of medications, are more likely than younger people to need information on side effects and interactions between medications, yet a recent consumer study on consumers' reception of printed DTC advertisements found that older Americans are less likely than their younger counterparts to find educational value in printed DTC advertisements. Specifically, American adults of 60 and above were more likely to say that such advertisements "never" tell them what the advertised product is for, and were more likely to state that printed DTC advertisements do not clearly convey that the advertised product is available only via prescription (Foley, 2000).

Moreover, preliminary research suggests that exposure to DTC advertisements may not equate with being better educated about one's relative risk of developing certain diseases that affect people from all demographic groups. A recent content analysis of printed DTC advertisements appearing in popular magazines during 1998 and 1999 suggested that rather than helping to eliminate common health misperceptions, the advertisements tend to reinforce misleading gender and racial stereotypes about the types of conditions that afflict different populations (Cline & Young, 2004). Of the advertisements featuring women only, Cline and Young (2004) found that nearly half focused on women in their reproductive capacity, reinforcing the notion that women's health is synonymous with women's reproductive health. Women also dominated advertisements for psychiatric medications. Two thirds of psychiatric advertisements featured only women. Conversely, two thirds of cardiovascular-related advertisements featured only men, despite the fact that cardiovascular disease is the number one killer of both men and women (Anderson & Smith, 2005). Moreover, although cardiovascular disease is the leading cause of death for whites, African Americans, and

Latinos alike (Anderson & Smith, 2005), every single advertisement for a cardiovascular-related product exclusively featured white people (Cline & Young, 2004). Thus, preliminary evidence on DTCA suggests that certain demographic groups are more likely to be targeted than others. A number of critical questions remain unanswered: Does this targeting happen via broadcast DTCA as well as via printed DTC advertisements? Do various groups of Americans respond differently to DTCA?

GENDER DISPARITIES IN U.S. MEDICINE

Despite some successful attempts to combat gender-based disparities in medical care over the last several decades, glaring gaps in medical care continue to exist in the United States. One way of narrowing these gaps is by better educating women patients about their risks of disease, and emphasizing the importance of taking an active role in their own care (Krupat, Irish, & Kasten, 1999). To the extent that DTC advertisements actually reach vulnerable populations, educate them about their relative risk of developing certain under-diagnosed conditions (like cardiovascular disease) and about potential treatments for these conditions, and facilitate patient-physician communication, DTC advertisements have the potential to reduce gender-based disparities in U.S. health care. If, however, DTC advertisements simply reproduce gender-based stereotypes about disease and medical care, it follows that women could be more susceptible to the negative effects of DTC advertisements described by the critics than men are.

One potential source of gender differences in medical care that could be affected by exposure to DTC advertisements is the misconception (shared by physicians, as well as by the general public) that certain diseases that affect all demographic groups such as cardiovascular disease, lung cancer, and kidney failure are not a threat to women (Gijsbers van Wijk, van Vliet, & Kolk, 1996). Cardiovascular disease, for example, is the number one killer of both American men *and* women (Anderson & Smith, 2005), but due, in part, to the complete lack of women represented in a number of high-profile clinical trials of cardiovascular disease treatments in the early 1980s (Carnes, 1999) and the continued underrepresentation of women in cardiovascular-related clinical trials (Bandyopadhyay, Bayer, & O'Mahony, 2001), the public (Erblich, Bovbjerg, Norman, Valdimarsdottir, & Montgomery, 2000) and physicians alike (Carnes, 1999) tend to share the mistaken belief that heart disease is a predominantly male phenomenon. This misapprehension is further institutionalized as a result of cardiovascular advertisements appearing in medical journals that overwhelmingly feature more images of male than female patients suffering from heart disease (Ahmed, Grace, Stelfox, Cheung, & Cheung, 2004; Leppard, Maile Ogletree, & Wallen, 1993). Physicians are less likely to educate women adequately about their risk factors for such conditions than they are men because physicians may not perceive women's actual level of risk (Yawn, Wollan, Jacobsen, Fryer, & Roger, 2004) and as a result, may not properly evaluate them. Given that two thirds of the printed DTC advertisements about heart-disease medication feature men exclusively (Cline & Young, 2004), these DTC advertisements are likely to reproduce the gender disparities in the propensity to seek and receive treatment for heart disease.

Another source of gender disparities in medical care emanates from physicians misreading women's presentation of symptoms, either because women present different symptoms than men for the same conditions (Charney, 2002; Jneid & Thacker, 2001; Philpott, Boynton, Feder, & Hemingway, 2001), or because they present in a different manner (e.g., emotionally rather than reservedly) than men (Elderkin-Thompson & Waitzkin, 1999). Put another way, male patients are unmarked; their symptoms and styles of presentation are taken as the standard because of men's dominance in clinical trials (Carnes, 1999) and medical textbooks (Curry, 2001). Women's symptoms and styles of presentation, then, are marked, and sometimes unrecognizable if they deviate from that of the "typical" male patient (Bickell et al., 1992). Physicians' misreading of women's presentation of symptoms leads to misdiagnosis of either the severity of the condition or of the condition itself, often with severe consequences (Munch, 2004). Examples of this in literature on the subject include women who present with symptoms of bladder disease frequently being diagnosed with the psychiatric condition of somatization disorder, resulting in mistreatment of the disease (Webster, 1993); physicians prescribing activity restrictions to female patients more readily than to male patients with equivalent symptoms and demographic profiles (Safran, Rogers, & Tarlov, 1997); women with kidney disease receiving fewer kidney transplantations than men (Evans, Blagg, & Bryan, 1981; Held, Pauly, Bovbjerg, Newmann, & Salvatierra, 1988); and the widely argued, although contested finding[1] that women with cardiovascular disease are often treated less aggressively than men (e.g., Bertoni, Bonds, Lovato, Goff, & Brancati, 2004; Di Cecco, Patel, & Upshur, 2002; Miller, Byington, Hunninghake, Pitt, & Furberg, 2000; Rathore, Chen, Wang, Radford, Vaccarino, & Krumholz, 2001; Thurau, 1997). To the extent that women become better educated about their conditions through DTC advertisements than men do, they should be better equipped to negotiate appropriate diagnoses and treatment from their health care providers.

Women of color and of lower socioeconomic status (SES) in the United States are doubly disadvantaged in terms of medical interventions and outcomes compared to white men (e.g., Rothenberg, Pearson, Zwanziger, & Mukamel, 2004; Schulman et al., 1999). Minority women in particular tend to be underrepresented as patients in medical textbooks (Curry, 2001), and lower class women discuss less and spend less time with their physicians than do either men or middle class women (Epstein, Taylor, & Seage, 1985; Roter, Lipkin, & Korsgaard, 1991). Moreover, African Americans and Latinos are at a higher risk than whites for many serious diseases, including cardiovascular disease (Yancy, 2004) and HIV (Dean, Steele, Satcher, & Nakashima, 2005), yet, as patients they tend to have fewer educational resources at their disposal (Redman, 1999). Finally, functional health literacy is a serious issue in the African American and other ethnic and racial communities (Georges, Bumes Bolton, & Bennett, 2004), communities historically characterized by socioeconomic disadvantage. If they target a relatively well-educated audience, DTC advertisements could benefit white women more than Latinas or African American women, thus reproducing racial disparities in health care.

RESEARCH QUESTIONS

In light of the potential health impact of DTC advertisements on women in general, and on women from lower SES and minority groups in particular, this study poses a number of unanswered questions. With respect to exposure to DTCA, this study asks: What types of sources do Americans use to gather health care information? Are American women more likely than their male counterparts to have been exposed to a DTC advertisement? Are minority women and women of lower SES equally likely to have been exposed to DTCA as their white, better educated, and wealthier counterparts?

With respect to taking action as a result of seeing or hearing a DTC advertisement, this study asks: Who is more likely to consult a physician as a result of exposure to a DTC advertisement—men or women; minorities or whites; people of lower or higher SES?

With respect to physician actions as a result of a DTCA-induced visit, this study asks: What type of actions do physicians take as a result of DTCA-related visits? Do these actions vary according to patients' gender? What type of new diagnoses do DTC advertisements help to generate? Do these new diagnoses differ according to patients' gender? Finally, how often has DTCA led to new diagnoses of cardiovascular disease in women, a disease often framed as a male problem? To wit, how often has DTCA led to new diagnoses of psychiatric disorders in women, diagnoses traditionally given more often to women than men (Hohmann, 1989)?

DATA

The data are from a nationally representative, cross-sectional telephone survey conducted between July 9, 2001, and January 16, 2002, with 3,000 adult participants. The survey, "The Public Health Impact of Direct-to-Consumer Advertising of Prescription Drugs," was designed by a group of researchers from Harvard University/Massachusetts General Hospital and Harris Interactive in order to gauge public attitudes and health practices associated with DTCA. Participants were chosen using random-digit dialing and random-household-member selection procedures; the response rate was 53% (Weissman et al., 2003). All analyses were done on weighted data that reflect the U.S. population in 2001, based on estimates from the March 2001 Current Population Survey.

One major shortcoming of the "Public Health Impact" survey is that while it asked a series of questions about physician visits prompted by DTC advertisements, it did not ask respondents about physician visits *not* prompted by DTC advertisements. Without a control group, it is not possible to infer, for example, whether new diagnoses generated in DTCA-induced visits were the result of the advertisements only, or whether those same new diagnoses would have been generated in physician visits prompted by other factors (Bodenheimer, 2003). While this is indeed a drawback, Weissman and colleagues (2003) pointed out that due to the ubiquitous nature of DTC advertisements, and the myriad reasons patients tend to give for scheduling appointments with physicians, identifying a pure experimental group (patients who *only* scheduled appointments as a result of seeing or hearing a DTC advertisement) and a pure control group (patients who were *not at all* influenced to schedule an appointment by any DTC advertisements they had seen or heard over the last year) would be virtually impossible.

ANALYTICAL STRATEGY

As explained under the section "Research Questions," the analyses sought to answer three broad research questions:

1. Which groups of Americans are more likely to be exposed to DTCA?
2. Which groups are more likely to schedule a physician visit due to exposure to DTCA?
3. What types of actions do physicians take as the result of a DTCA-related visit?

For each of these broad questions we began by testing gender differences (e.g., were women more likely to be exposed to DTCA than were men?). Where gender differences existed, we restricted our analyses to women only, and tested differences between groups of women based on race or ethnicity, education, and household income (e.g., were wealthier, white, or better educated women more likely than their poorer, minority, or less-educated counterparts to be exposed to DTCA?).

Bivariate relationships (such as the relationship between respondents' gender and their sources of health information, or the relationship between respondents' gender and their exposure to a DTC advertisement) were tested using the chi-square statistic and are presented, for ease of interpretation, in figure form in the body of the chapter. Multivariate relationships were tested using logistic-regression analyses that control for multiple factors that may affect respondents' likelihood of having been exposed to a DTC advertisement, their likelihood of responding to a DTC advertisement by scheduling a physician visit, and the likelihood that their physician took various actions as a result of the visit. In the multivariate analyses, we report the odds ratios of the regression models, or the ratio of the odds of an event occurring in one group to the odds of it occurring in another group. Odds ratios greater than 1 indicate a positive relationship between an independent variable (e.g., female gender) and the dependent variable (e.g., exposure to DTCA), or, in the preceding example, a greater likelihood that women have been exposed to a DTC advertisement than men have. Odds ratios of less than 1 indicate a negative relationship between an independent variable and a dependent variable, or, in the preceding example, a lower likelihood that women have been exposed to a DTC advertisement than men have. While key multivariate results are discussed in the body of the chapter, full results for each of the multivariate analyses appear in the appendices located at the back of this book.

RESULTS

Table 1 provides descriptive statistics for the variables used in the analyses.

TABLE 1. Descriptive statistics for variables in analyses.

	%
Sex (*n* = 3,000)	
Female	52.0
Male	48.0
Race (*n* = 2,953)	
White	76.3
African American/Black	12.2
Other	11.5
Ethnicity (*n* = 2,966)	
Latino/Latina	10.6
Education (*n* = 2,986)	
No high school diploma	11.1
High school graduate/some college	65.7
College graduate	23.2
Household income (*n* = 2,689)	
< $25,000/year	27.5
$25,000 to $49,999/year	35.3
$50,000/year and above	37.2
Age (*n* = 3,000)	
18–34	32.0
35–64	51.3
65+	16.7
Gather health information from:	
Physicians (*n* = 2,942)	66.7
Family/Friends (*n* = 2,980)	57.3
Advertising (*n* = 2,988)	57.1
Pamphlets in doctors' offices (*n* = 2,978)	49.5
Magazines (*n* = 2,979)	46.6
TV/Radio (*n* = 2,980)	46.3
Pharmacists (*n* = 2,967)	35.2
Internet (*n* = 2,994)	23.5
Saw or heard DTCA in last 12 months (*n* = 2,987)	83.6
DTCA ever prompted you to speak to doctor (*n* = 2,601)	40.7
As the result of a DTCA-induced visit:	
Doctor prescribed drug (*n* = 953)	72.9
Doctor referred you to a specialist (*n* = 952)	32.6
Doctor suggested change in diet/exercise (*n* = 951)	52.0
Doctor suggested over-the-counter drug (*n* = 952)	19.1
Doctor ordered laboratory test (*n* = 951)	57.3
Doctor suggested you quit smoking (*n* = 943)	33.9

(*continued on next page*)

TABLE 1. (continued)

	%
Have regular doctor you go to when sick (n = 2,991)	80.0
Have health-insurance coverage (n = 2,991)	83.4
Have prescription-drug coverage (n = 2,924)	76.1
Regularly take any prescription drugs (n = 2,992)	49.5
Self-rated health (n = 2,987)	
Excellent	21.4
Very good	30.5
Good	31.4
Fair	12.2
Poor	4.6
Previously diagnosed with:	
Diabetes (n = 2,992)	7.5
Depression (n = 2,992)	12.4
Arthritis (n = 2,987)	19.8
Cancer (n = 2,994)	6.4
Heart disease (n = 2,986)	7.6
Hypertension/High blood pressure (n = 2,988)	22.9
High cholesterol (n = 2,975)	20.1
Stroke (n = 2,995)	2.6
Allergies (n = 2,985)	26.5
Asthma (n = 2,993)	11.9
Anxiety (n = 2,989)	10.6
Other emotional/mental illness (n = 2,986)	2.2
Other chronic condition (n = 2,972)	15.3
Heart disease, hypertension, high cholesterol, or stroke (n = 2,996)	35.3
Depression, Anxiety, or other emotional/mental illness (n = 2,996)	17.0

The top three sources respondents used to gather health information were physicians (66.7%), family or friends (57.3%), and advertisements (57.1%). The vast majority (83.6%) of respondents had been exposed to DTCA during the past year. Of those who had seen a DTC advertisement, 2 in 5 went on to consult a physician about an advertisement. The most common physician actions taken as the result of a DTCA-induced visit were to prescribe the patient a drug (72.9%), to order a laboratory test (57.3%), and to suggest the patient change her or his diet or exercise routine (52.0%). Approximately half of respondents (49.5%) reported regularly taking a prescription drug.

SOURCES OF HEALTH INFORMATION

Figure 1 presents information on respondents' sources of health information, broken down by patients' gender.

Notably, women reported using each and every source of information to gather health care information more often than men did, a finding that suggests that women are somewhat more vigilant and concerned than men are about staying apprised of the latest health care information. This is not entirely surprising, given that women are frequently responsible for managing not just their own health care, but also the health and health

FIGURE 1. Percentage who regularly use various sources to gain health information by gender.

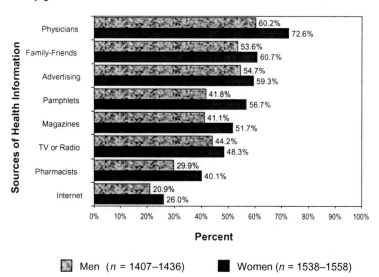

Note. All are significant at $p < .05$.

care utilization of their families (Weisman, 1987). If women desire, and make an effort to be better informed than men about health care choices, a finding supported by some recent studies (Arora and McHorney, 2000; Stewart et al., 2004), they may be more likely than men to pay attention to DTC advertisements and to respond to them, especially given the fact that women use more health services than men do (Green & Pope, 1999).

EXPOSURE TO DIRECT-TO-CONSUMER ADVERTISEMENTS

Figure 2 depicts the percentage of respondents (broken down according to patients' gender) who were exposed to DTCA in the 12 months prior to the survey. While the vast majority of both men and women had seen a direct-to-consumer advertisement in the year prior to the survey, women were slightly more likely to have seen such an advertisement than men were.

FIGURE 2. Percentage who saw/heard DTCA in the last 12 months by gender.

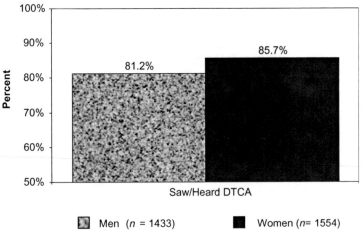

Men (*n* = 1433)   Women (*n*= 1554)

Note. X^2 = 11.09, *df* = 1, p < .01.

There were significant differences in exposure to DTCA among women, based on race or ethnicity, education level, and household income (see Figure 3). More than 9 out of 10 white women, college-educated women, and women with household incomes of $50,000 per year or more had seen or heard a DTC advertisement in the year prior to the survey. Latinas, women without a high school diploma, and women from households with an annual income of less than $25,000 were particularly less likely to have seen a DTC advertisement. The results of the multivariate analyses that controlled for multiple factors that may have affected respondents' likelihood of having been exposed to a DTC advertisement, and their ability to remember having seen such an advertisement, appear in Appendix A. Once other factors that might have affected exposure were taken into account, the patterns reported above continued to hold: Women, those with more education, and those with higher household incomes were more likely to report having seen or heard a DTC advertisement than were men, those with less education, and those with lower household incomes,

FIGURE 3. Percentage who saw/heard a DTC ad in the last 12 months by race/ethnicity,[a] income,[b] and education.[c]

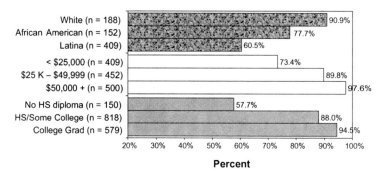

[a] X^2 = 120.26, df = 2, p < .001.
[b] X^2 = 120.85, df = 2, p < .001.
[c] X^2 = 147.60, df = 2, p < .001.

respectively. African Americans and Latinas were significantly less likely to have seen or heard such an advertisement than were whites. In the women-only multivariate analysis of likelihood of exposure to DTCA (see Appendix B), the same trends exist (i.e., higher socio-economic status was related to a higher likelihood of having seen an advertisement in the last 12 months; minority status was related to a lower likelihood).

PHYSICIAN CONTACT AS A RESULT OF A DIRECT-TO-CONSUMER ADVERTISEMENT

Among those respondents who reported having seen a DTC advertisement, women were more likely than men to report having consulted a physician as the result of the advertisement (see Figure 4). Once other factors that might have affected respondents' likelihood of contacting a physician due to a DTC advertisement were taken into account, being a woman, being African

FIGURE 4. DTCA ever prompted them to speak to a doctor by gender (only asked of those who had heard/seen or been told about a DTC ad).

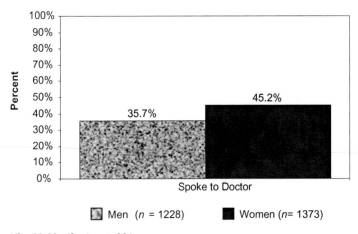

Men (*n* = 1228)   Women (*n*= 1373)

Note. X^2 = 23.69, *df* = 1, p < .001.

FIGURE 5. DTCA ever prompted them to speak to a doctor by race/ethnicity,[a] income,[b] and education[c] (women only; only asked of those who had heard/seen or been told about a DTC ad).

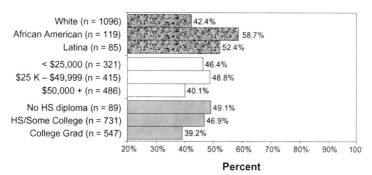

[a] X^2 = 15.63, df = 2, p < .001.
[b] X^2 = 6.56, df = 2, p < .05.
[c] X^2 = 7.16, df = 2, p < .05.

American, and having fewer years of schooling were all associated with a greater likelihood of contacting a physician due to a DTC advertisement. In analyses restricted to women only, African Americans, Latinas, the less educated, and those with lower incomes were more likely to contact a physician due to the content of a DTC advertisement than were their white, more educated, wealthier counterparts (see Figure 5). Being African American and less educated continued to be significantly associated with a higher likelihood of contacting a physician due to DTCA exposure (see Appendix B) once other factors that might have affected respondents' likelihood of contacting a physician due to DTCA were taken into account.

PHYSICIAN ACTIONS TAKEN AS A RESULT OF A DTCA-INDUCED VISIT

Figure 6 presents physicians' actions taken during DTCA-induced visits, broken down according to the patients' gender.

FIGURE 6. Percentage who reported doctor took various actions as a result of a DTCA-induced visit by gender.

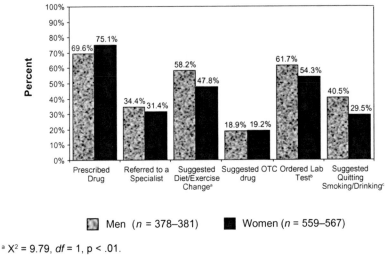

Men (n = 378–381)   Women (n = 559–567)

ᵃ X^2 = 9.79, df = 1, p < .01.
ᵇ X^2 = 5.11, df = 1, p < .05.
ᶜ X^2 = 12.08, df = 1, p < .01.

Physicians prescribed a drug, referred to a specialist, and suggested an over-the-counter drug as frequently for women as they did for men who came to see them as the result of a DTC advertisement (see Figure 6). Physicians were significantly less likely to order a laboratory test or to suggest a lifestyle change for women than they were for men. This same pattern emerged when controlling for potential confounding factors (see Appendix C).[2] While the data do not allow us to determine whether physician responses were appropriate, they are nonetheless suggestive. The analyses reported in Appendix C suggest that physicians confronted by patients who schedule appointments due to exposure to DTC advertisements are less willing to broach certain subjects (such as lifestyle changes) with their female patients, and that physicians treat their female patients less aggressively than they do their male patients, with respect to ordering laboratory tests. The latter

FIGURE 7. Top five new diagnoses due to DTCA-induced visit by gender.

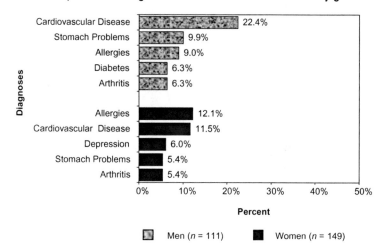

finding fits into the body of literature that finds women patients are treated less aggressively for certain conditions than male patients are (Bertoni et al., 2004; Bongard et al., 2004; Herold et al., 1997; Hochleitner, 2000; Kim, Hofer, & Kerr, 2003; Munch, 2004; Raine, 2000; Rathore et al., 2001; Vodopiutz, Poller, Schneider, Lalouschek, Menz, & Stollberger, 2002).

Figure 7 presents the top five new diagnoses (broken down according the patients' gender) given to respondents as the result of a DTCA-induced visit. Of the male patients who received a diagnosis for a previously undiagnosed condition during a DTCA-induced visit, the number one new diagnosis was cardiovascular disease,[3] at 22.4%. The top new diagnosis given to female patients was allergies, at 12.1%.

Figure 8 compares the percentage of new cardiovascular disease and psychiatric disorder[4] diagnoses (broken down according to patients' gender) generated by DTCA-induced visits.

Men were more than twice as likely as women to receive a new diagnosis of cardiovascular disease due to a DTC advertisement, and women

FIGURE 8. DTCA-related new diagnoses—cardiovascular disease and psychiatric disorders by gender.

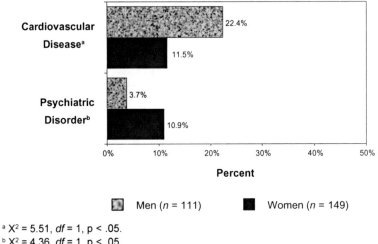

ᵃ X^2 = 5.51, df = 1, p < .05.
ᵇ X^2 = 4.36, df = 1, p < .05.

were nearly 3 times as likely to receive a psychiatric diagnosis as men. The survey was, unfortunately, not adjusted according to how many DTCA-induced visits respondents scheduled and attended. Given the fact that women utilize health care services more frequently than men do (Green & Pope, 1999), women should be more likely than men to receive all diagnoses, because women have more chances to receive diagnoses. Thus, women's greater use of health care in general may help to explain female respondents' greater likelihood of receiving a psychiatric diagnosis. Nevertheless, women's more frequent health care utilization makes it even more remarkable that they are just half as likely as men to receive a new diagnosis of cardiovascular disease as the result of a DTCA-related visit. These findings on the types of new diagnoses generated strongly suggest that the type of conditions that DTC advertisements target differs according to gender, a finding supported by a recent content analysis of printed DTC advertisements (Cline & Young, 2004).

Discussion

In summary, women are more likely to turn to a variety of sources for health information than men are. Women are more likely to have seen a DTC advertisement, and are more likely to have consulted a doctor as the result of an advertisement than men are. Women from minority groups and women of lower socioeconomic status are less likely to have seen an advertisement, but African American and less-educated women are more likely to speak to a doctor as the result of a DTC advertisement than white or more-educated women are. This suggests, ironically, that groups of women with the greatest health-information needs and with a greater likelihood of actually scheduling a physician visit as the result of exposure to a DTC advertisement are less likely to see such advertisements, and thus gain an educational benefit from them. Moreover, physicians are less likely to take certain actions with women than with men as the result of a DTCA-induced visit, and the frequency with which conditions are diagnosed due to DTCA-induced visits differs according to the patients' gender. While the data do not allow an evaluation of appropriateness of these interventions, they certainly suggest the gendered content of DTC advertisements.

Rather than narrowing existing gaps in U.S. health care by alerting consumers to their likelihood of developing underdiagnosed health conditions, DTC advertisements appear to reinforce existing gender-, race-, and class-based disparities in care. For example, they seem to reinforce the inaccurate notion that cardiovascular disease is a predominantly male phenomenon, given the lower rate at which women who schedule physician visits due to DTCA go on to receive a new diagnosis of CVD compared to men. Furthermore, DTCA appears to have the potential to narrow health information disparities between white and African American women, and between better educated and less-educated women, given that both African American women and less-educated women are more likely to respond to DTC advertisements than their white and better educated female counterparts are. Nevertheless, DTCA's potential for narrowing the health information gap between different groups of women is unlikely to be realized, given that African American women and less-educated women are significantly less likely to be exposed to DTCA than white women or more educated women are, due to pharmaceutical companies' targeting of certain demographic groups deemed more likely to buy products than others (Turow, 1997).

Finally, it is a testament to the power of existing cultural schemas that (1) pharmaceutical companies have not highlighted women's risk of cardiovascular disease to the degree that they have highlighted men's risks, and (2) that they have neglected targeting African American women and less-educated women to the same degree that they have targeted white women and better educated women. Given that women are as likely to die from cardiovascular disease as men, and given that African American women and less-educated women are actually more likely to respond to a DTC advertisement by scheduling a physician visit than white women or better educated women are, neglecting these groups likely represents a poor business decision. Clearly, even marketing executives have trouble breaking through our socially constructed notions of who is likely to suffer from various diseases, and which groups of Americans are more likely to contact physicians as a result of direct-to-consumer advertisements, and are thus more likely to buy advertised prescription drugs.

References

Ahmed, S., Grace, S., Stelfox, H, Cheung, G., & Cheung, A. (2004). Gender bias in cardiovascular advertisements. *Journal of Evaluation in Clinical Practice, 10*(4), 531–538.

Aikin, K., Swasy, J., & Braman, A. (2004). *Patient and physician attitudes and behaviors associated with DTC promotion of prescription drugs* (Summary of FDA survey research results). U.S. Food and Drug Administration, Center for Drug Evaluation and Research, Rockville, MD.

Anderson, R., & Smith, B. (2005). "Deaths: Leading causes for 2002." National Center for Health Statistics. *National Vital Statistics Reports No. 53*(17), 1–92.

Arora, N., & McHorney, C. (2000). Patient preferences for medical decision-making: Who really wants to participate? *Medical Care, 38*(3), 335–341.

Bandyopadhyay, S., Bayer, A., & O'Mahony, M. (2001). Age and gender bias in statin trials. *Quarterly Journal of Medicine, 94*(3), 127–132.

Bell, R., Kravitz, R., & Wilkes, M. (1999). Direct-to-consumer prescription drug advertising and the public. *Journal of General Internal Medicine, 14*(11), 651–657.

Bell, R., Wilkes, M., & Kravitz, R. (1999). Advertisement-induced prescription drug requests—Patients' anticipated reactions to a physician who refuses. *Journal of Family Practice, 48*(6), 446–452.

Bertoni, A., Bonds, D., Lovato, J., Goff, D., & Brancati, F. (2004). Sex disparities in procedure use for acute myocardial infarction in the United States, 1995 to 2001. *American Heart Journal, 147*(6), 1054–1060.

Bickell, N., Pieper, K., Lee, K., Mark, D., Glower, D., Pryor, D., et al. (1992). Referral patterns for coronary artery disease treatment: Gender bias or good clinical judgment? *Annals of Internal Medicine, 116*(10), 791–797.

Blum, M., Slade, M., Boden, D., Cabin, H., & Caulin-Glaser, T. (2004). Examination of gender bias in the evaluation and treatment of angina pectoris by cardiologists. *American Journal of Cardiology, 93*(6), 765–767.

Bodenheimer, T. (2003). Perspective: Two advertisements for TV drug ads. *Health Affairs (Web Exclusives* Suppl. W3), 112–115.

Bongard, V., Grenier, O., Ferrières, J., Danchin, N., Cantet, C., Amelineau, E., et al. (2004). Drug prescriptions and referral to cardiac rehabilitation after acute coronary events: Comparison between men and women in the French PREVENIR Survey. *International Journal of Cardiology, 93*(2–3), 217–223.

Brownfield, E., Bernhardt, J., Phan, J., Williams, M., & Parker, R. (2004). Direct-to-consumer drug advertisements on network television: An exploration of quantity, frequency, and placement. *Journal of Health Communication, 9*(6), 491–497.

Calfee, J. (2002). Public policy issues in direct-to-consumer advertising of prescription drugs. *Journal of Public Policy & Marketing, 21*(2), 174–193.

Carnes, M. (1999). Health care in the U.S.: Is there evidence for systematic gender bias? *Wisconsin Medical Journal, 98*(8), 15–25.

Charney, P. (2002). Presenting symptoms and diagnosis of coronary heart disease in women. *Journal of Cardiovascular Risk, 9*(6), 303–307.

Cline, R., & Young, H. (2004). Marketing drugs, marketing health care relationships: A content analysis of visual cues in direct-to-consumer prescription drug advertising. *Health Communication, 16*(2), 131–157.

Conrad, P., & Leiter, V. (2004). Medicalization, markets and consumers. *Journal of Health & Social Behavior, 45*(Suppl. 1), 158–176.

Courtenay, W., McCreary, D., & Merighi, J. (2002). Gender and ethnic differences in health beliefs and behaviors. *Journal of Health Psychology, 7*(3), 219–231.

Curry, M. (2001). Patterns of race and gender representation in health assessment textbooks. *Journal of National Black Nurses' Association, 12*(2), 3035.

Dean, H., Steele, C., Satcher, A., & Nakashima, A. (2005). HIV/AIDS among minority races and ethnicities in the United States, 1999–2003. *Journal of the National Medical Association, 97*(Suppl. 7), 5S–12S.

Di Cecco, R., Patel, U., & Upshur, R. (2002). Is there a clinically significant gender bias in post-myocardial infarction pharmacological management in the older (>60) population of a primary care practice? *BMC Family Practice, 3*, 8.

Elderkin-Thompson, V., & Waitzkin, H. (1999). Differences in clinical communication by gender. *Journal of General Internal Medicine, 14*(2), 112–121.

Epstein, A., Taylor, W., & Seage, G. III. (1985). Effects of patients' socioeconomic status and physicians' training and practice on patient-doctor communication. *American Journal of Medicine, 78*(1), 101–116.

Erblich, J., Bovbjerg, D., Norman, C., Valdimarsdottir, H., & Montgomery, G. (2000). It won't happen to me: Lower perception of heart disease risk among women with family histories of breast cancer. *Preventive Medicine, 31*(6), 714–721.

Evans, R., Blagg, C., & Bryan, F., Jr. (1981). Implications for health care policy. A social and demographic profile of hemodialysis patients in the United States. *Journal of the American Medical Association, 245*(5), 487–491.

Foley, L. (2000). The medication information gap: Older consumers in the void between direct-to-consumer advertising and professional care. *Generations, 24*(4), 49–54.

Gahart, M., Duhamel, L., Dievler, A., & Price, R. (2003). Examining the FDA's oversight of direct-to-consumer advertising. *Health Affairs* (*Web Exclusives* Suppl. W3), 120–123.

Georges, C., Bumes Bolton, L., & Bennett, C. (2004). Functional health literacy: An issue in African-American and other ethnic and racial communities. *Journal of National Black Nurses' Association*, 15(1), 1–4.

Gijsbers van Wijk, C., van Vliet, K., & Kolk, A. (1996). Gender perspectives and quality of care: Towards appropriate and adequate health care for women. *Social Science & Medicine, 43*(5), 707–720.

Green, C., & Pope, C. (1999). Gender, psychosocial factors and the use of medical services: A longitudinal analysis. *Social Science & Medicine, 48*(10), 1363–1372.

Held, P., Pauly, M., Bovbjerg, R., Newmann, J., & Salvatierra, O. Jr. (1988). Access to kidney transplantation: Has the United States eliminated income and racial differences? *Archives of Internal Medicine, 148*(12), 2594–2600.

Herold, A., Riker, A., Warner, E., Woodard, L., Brownlee, H., Jr., Pencev, D., et al. (1997). Evidence of gender bias in patients undergoing flexible sigmoidoscopy. *Cancer Detection & Prevention, 21*(2), 141–147.

Hochleitner, M. (2000). Coronary heart disease: Sexual bias in referral for coronary angiogram. How does it work in a state-run health system? *Journal of Women's Health & Gender-Based Medicine, 9*(1), 29–34.

Hohmann, A. (1989). Gender bias in psychotropic drug prescribing in primary care. *Medical Care, 27*(5), 478–490.

Holmer, A. (1999). Direct-to-consumer prescription drug advertising builds bridges between patients and physicians. *Journal of the American Medical Association, 281*(4), 380–382.

Holmer, A. (2002). Direct-to-consumer advertising—Strengthening our health care system. *New England Journal of Medicine, 346*(7), 526–528.

IMS Health. (2006). *Total U.S. promotional spending by type, 2005.* Retrieved September 13, 2006, from http://www.imshealth.com/ims/ portal/front/articleC/0,2777,6599_9285_1004963,00.html

Jneid, H., & Thacker, H. (2001). Coronary artery disease in women: Different, often undertreated. *Cleveland Clinic Journal of Medicine, 68*(5), 441–448.

Kim, C., Hofer, T., & Kerr, E. (2003). Review of evidence and explanations for suboptimal screening and treatment of dyslipidemia in women—A conceptual model. *Journal of General Internal Medicine, 18*(10), 854–863.

Kravitz, R., Epstein, R., Feldman, M., Franz, C., Azari, R., Wilkes, et al. (2005). Influence of patients' requests for direct-to-consumer advertised antidepressants: A randomized controlled trial. *Journal of the American Medical Association, 293*(16), 1995–2002.

Krieger, L. (1998, December 7). What's right about drug ads. *New York Times*, p. A25.

Krupat, E., Irish, J., Kasten, L., Freund, K., Burns, R., Moskowitz, M., et al. (1999). Patient assertiveness and physician decision-making among older breast cancer patients. *Social Science & Medicine, 49*(4), 449–457.

Laurence, L., & Weinhouse, B. (1997). *Outrageous practices: How gender bias threatens women's health.* New Brunswick, NJ: Rutgers University Press.

Leppard, W., Maile Ogletree, S., & Wallen, E. (1993). Gender stereotyping in medical advertising: Much ado about something? *Sex Roles, 29*, 829–838.

Lyles, A. (2002). Direct marketing of pharmaceuticals to consumers. *Annual Review of Public Health, 23*, 73–91.

Mansfield, P., & Mintzes, B. (2003). Direct-to-consumer advertising is more profitable if it is misleading. *New Zealand Medical Journal, 116*(1182), U610.

Mansfield, P., Mintzes, B., Richards, D., & Toop, L. (2005). Direct to consumer advertising is at the crossroads of competing pressures from industry and health needs. *British Medical Journal, 330*, 5–6.

Miller, M., Byington, R., Hunninghake, D., Pitt, B., & Furberg, C. (2000). Sex bias and underutilization of lipid-lowering therapy in patients with coronary artery disease at academic medical centers in the United States and Canada. *Archives of Internal Medicine, 160*(3), 343–347.

Mintzes, B., Barer, M., Kravitz, R., Bassett, K., Lexchin, J., Kazanjian, A., et al. (2003). How does direct-to-consumer advertising (DTCA) affect prescribing? A survey in primary care environments with and without legal DTCA. *Canadian Medical Association Journal, 169*(5), 405–412.

Munch, S. (2004). Gender-biased diagnosing of women's medical complaints: Contributions of feminist thought, 1970–1995. *Women & Health, 40*(1), 101–121.

Murray, E., Lo, B., Pollack, L., Donelan, K., & Lee, K. (2004). Direct-to-consumer advertising: Public perceptions of its effects on health behaviors, health care, and the doctor-patient relationship. *Journal of the American Board of Family Practice, 17*(1), 6–18.

Perri, M. III, Shinde, S., & Banavali, R. (1999). The past, present, and future of direct-to-consumer prescription drug advertising. *Clinical Therapeutics, 21*(10), 1798–1811.

Philpott, S., Boynton, P., Feder, G., & Hemingway, H. (2001). Gender differences in descriptions of angina symptoms and health problems immediately prior to angiography: The ACRE study. *Social Science & Medicine, 52*(10), 1565–1575.

Prevention Magazine. (2001). *International survey on wellness and consumer reactions to DTC advertising of Rx drugs: 2000–2001.* Emmaus, PA: Rodale Press.

Raine, R. (2000). Does gender bias exist in the use of specialist health care? *Journal of Health Services Research & Policy, 5*(4), 237–249.

Rathore, S., Chen, J., Wang, Y., Radford, M., Vaccarino, V., & Krumholz, H. (2001). Sex differences in cardiac catheterization—The role of physician gender. *Journal of the American Medical Association, 286*(22), 2849–2856.

Redman, B. (1999). *Women's health needs in patient education.* New York: Springer Publishing Company.

Roger, V., Farkouh, M., Weston, S., Reeder, G., Jacobsen, S., Zinsmeister, et al. (2000). Sex differences in evaluation and outcome of unstable angina. *Journal of the American Medical Association, 283*(5), 646–652.

Rosenthal, M., Berndt, E., Donohue, J., Frank, R., & Epstein, A. (2002). Promotion of prescription drugs to consumers. *New England Journal of Medicine, 346*(7), 498–505.

Roter, D., Lipkin, M. Jr., & Korsgaard, A. (1991). Sex differences in patients' and physicians' communication during primary care medical visits. *Medical Care, 29*(11), 1083–1093.

Roter, D., & Hall, J. (1997). Gender differences in patient-physician communication. In J. Gallant, G. Puryear Keita, & R. Royak-Schaler (Eds.), *Health care for women: Psychological, social, and behavioral influences* (pp. 57–71). Washington, DC: American Psychological Association.

Rothenberg, B., Pearson, T., Zwanziger, J., & Mukamel, D. (2004). Explaining disparities in access to high-quality cardiac surgeons. *Annals of Thoracic Surgery, 78*(1), 18–24; discussion 24–25.

Safran, D., Rogers, W., & Tarlov, A. (1997). Gender differences in medical treatment: The case of physician-prescribed activity restrictions. *Social Science & Medicine, 45*(5), 711–722.

Schulman, K., Berlin, J., Harless, W., Kerner, J., Sistrunk, S., Gersh, B., et al. (1999). The effect of race and sex on physicians' recommendations for cardiac catheterization. *New England Journal of Medicine, 340*(8), 618–26.

Stanton, A., & Courtenay, W. (2004). Gender, stress, and health. In R. Rozensky, N. Johnson, C. Goodheart, & W. Hammond (Eds.), *Psychology builds a healthy world: Opportunities for research and practice* (pp. 105–135). Washington, DC: American Psychological Association.

Stewart, D., Abbey, S., Shnek, Z., Irvine, J., & Grace, S. (2004). Gender differences in health information needs and decisional preferences in patients recovering from an acute ischemic coronary event. *Psychosomatic Medicine, 66*(1), 42–48.

Thurau, R. (1997). Perceived gender bias in the treatment of cardiovascular disease. *Journal of Vascular Nursing, 15*(4), 124–127.

Turow, J. (1997). *Breaking up America: Advertisers and the new media world.* Chicago: University of Chicago Press.

U.S. General Accounting Office (2002). *Prescription Drugs: FDA oversight of direct-to-consumer advertising has limitations* (Rep. No. GAO-03-177). General Accounting Office, Washington, DC.

Vodopiutz, J., Poller, S., Schneider, B., Lalouschek, J., Menz, F., & Stollberger, C. (2002). Chest pain in hospitalized patients: Cause-specific and gender-specific differences. *Journal of Women's Health and Gender-Based Medicine, 11*(8), 719–727.

Vogel, R., Ramachandran, S., & Zachry, W. III. (2003). A 3-stage model for assessing the probable economic effects of direct-to-consumer advertising of pharmaceuticals. *Clinical Therapeutics, 25*(1), 309–329.

Waldron, I. (1997). Changing gender roles and gender differences in health behavior. In D. Gochman (Ed.), *Handbook of health behavior research: Personal and social determinants* (pp. 303–328). New York: Plenum Press.

Webster, D. (1993). Interstitial cystitis: Women at risk for psychiatric misdiagnosis. *AWHONNS Clinical Issues in Perinatal and Women's Health Nursing, 4*(2), 236–243.

Weisman, C. (1987). Communication between women and their health care providers: Research findings and unanswered questions. *Public Health Reports, 102*(Suppl.), 147–151.

Weissman, J., Blumenthal, D., Silk, A., Zapert, K., Newman, M., & Leitman, R. (2003). Consumers' reports on the health effects of direct-to-consumer drug advertising. *Health Affairs* (*Web Exclusives* Suppl. W3), 82–95.

Williams, D., & Collins, C. (1999). U.S. socioeconomic and racial differences in health: Patterns and explanations. In K. Charmaz & D. Paterniti (Eds.), *Health, illness, and healing: Society, social context, and self, an anthology* (pp. 349–376). Los Angeles: Roxbury Publishing.

Yancy, C. (2004). The prevention of heart failure in minority communities and discrepancies in health care delivery systems. *Medical Clinics of North America, 88*(5), 1347–1368.

Yawn, B., Wollan, P., Jacobsen, S., Fryer, G., & Roger, V. (2004). Identification of women's coronary heart disease and risk factors prior to first myocardial infarction. *Journal of Women's Health, 13*(10), 1087–1100.

ENDNOTES

1. The following are examples of studies that challenge the finding that women with cardiovascular disease are treated less aggressively: Blum, Slade, Boden, Cabin, and Caulin-Glaser (2004); Roger et al. (2000).
2. The number of women in the sample who reported various physician actions (including new diagnoses) as a result of a DTCA-related visit was insufficient to perform analyses on subgroups of women by education, income, and race or ethnicity.
3. Cardiovascular disease includes diagnoses of heart disease, hypertension, high cholesterol, stroke, vascular condition/clogged artery, and irregular heart beat.
4. Psychiatric disorder diagnoses include diagnoses of depression, anxiety, or "other mental health condition."

CHAPTER 4

COMPLEXITY AND CANCER:

THE MULTIPLE TEMPORALITIES
AND SPACES OF CANCER
IN RICHARD POWERS' *GAIN*

Lisa Diedrich

In their introduction to the volume *Complexities*, John Law and Annemarie Mol (2002) noted at the outset that, "[m]uch recent work in the sociology of science, history of technology, anthropology of medicine, feminism, and political philosophy has been a revolt against simplification" (p. 1). This "revolt against simplification" has meant that all of these interrelated and interdisciplinary fields have sought to demonstrate the complexity in the objects they study. For Law and Mol, attending to complexity means one is concerned about the way "things relate but don't add up," and their work seeks to discern but not order through simplification the chaos that exemplifies most experiences and events (p. 1). In their edited volume, Law and Mol (2002) have collected what they call "stories about what happens to complexity in practice" (p. 6). In fact, to signal the multiplicity of their approach, they explain that they have gathered together "stories about what happens to complexit*ies* in practic*es*" (p. 6).

In this essay, I consider Richard Powers' novel *Gain* (1998) as a story "about what happens to complexities in practices" that constitute one woman's experience of ovarian cancer in the fictional small town of Lacewood, Illinois, home of the Clare Corporation, a multinational conglomerate that manufactures everything from soap, to pharmaceuticals, to fertilizer. Powers shows the complexity of an individual woman's cancer by relating, but not adding up, the multiplicities that surround her experience of cancer in connection to larger social, economic, environmental, and political events. I want to investigate the multiplicities of cancer as presented in Powers' work, in order to ask how his novel helps us imagine and bring into being a complex understanding of health as an essential human right.

In the spirit of Law and Mol's work, I will offer a sketch of what I take to be *the multiple temporalities and spaces that literally make cancer* as demonstrated in Powers' novel. In particular, I will show the ways in which the novel *compounds rather than simplifies*[1] our understanding of cancer by bringing together in one story at least three temporalities of cancer: the time of disease, the time of illness, and the time of medicine. The novel also does this by framing the story in at least three spaces of cancer: the soap factory, the home, and the hospital.[2] Finally, I demonstrate that *Gain* offers several of what I call practices of witnessing—in and through suffering, the law, direct-action politics, and scientific research motivated by personal loss—for transforming the way we approach the experience and event of cancer. I use the term "practices of witnessing" instead of "forms of resistance" because it emphasizes that illness, as Annemarie Mol (2002) has argued, is enacted through practices. These practices take place on many levels from the micro to the macro: from the manipulation of genes and cells in individual bodies to the transformation of entire communities through endemic or epidemic diseases.

Illness is both an individual experience and a sociopolitical event; it is enacted over time and across spaces, from the inside out and the outside in. As Kelly Oliver (2001) has argued, the word "witnessing" has a double meaning; we witness what we have seen and what cannot be seen.[3] Witnessing is a historicopolitical and spiritual act. To witness is to engage in the presentation of historical evidence, to work for social justice, and to attempt to account for suffering and loss.

NOVELS AND THE COMPLEXITY OF CANCER

I want to begin by considering the form Powers has chosen for telling this story of complexity and cancer, and suggesting that writing itself and, in particular, the writing of novels, is, for Powers, another practice of witnessing. Unlike Arundhati Roy (1999), who has written that "[i]nstinct led me to set aside" literature in order to read "reports on drainage and irrigation" and to write political essays in support of the grassroots environmental-justice movement against the construction of Big Dams in India, Powers rather famously set aside science to write literature (p. 9).[4] On a very general level then, I am interested both in how people ascertain what narrative form they need to use, and in the dynamics of turning from one form to another. Roy begins by writing a novel, but discovers that this particular form cannot do what she thinks she needs it to do in the face of Big Dams and nuclear nationalism. For Powers, the movement is in the opposite direction, from scientific to literary narrative. Why does this matter? Or, more to the point, what does this turning from one form to another materialize, what does it bring into being in language?

In a recent essay in the *New York Times Book Review*, Rachel Donadio (2005) discussed Naipaul's claim in an interview in the same issue that "nonfiction is better suited than fiction to capturing the complexities of today's world" (p. 27). Donadio interviewed editors and others involved in book and magazine publishing, all of whom agree with Naipaul that, in the contemporary moment, fiction does not seem to have much "cultural currency" (p. 27). Donadio ends her essay by noting that

> [t]o date, no work of fiction has perfectly captured our historical
> moment the way certain novels captured the Gilded Age, or the
> Weimar Republic, or the cold war. Then again, it's still early.
> Nonfiction can keep up with the instant messenger culture; fic-
> tion takes its own sweet time. Even Tolstoy wrote *War and Peace*
> years after the Napoleonic Wars. Today the most compelling cre-
> ative energies seem directed at nonfiction. That is, until the next
> great novelist comes along to prove the naysayers wrong. Time, as
> Elizabeth Bishop once wrote, is nothing if not amenable. (p. 27)

In her essay, Donadio argued that writing novels requires a temporal
distance to events in the "real" world more than writing nonfiction does.
However, she neglected a second feature of the novel that undermines
her position: how its form is able to bring into being a different temporality, one that allows the reader a unique relationship to events in the
"real" world. It is this uniqueness that I believe Powers is trying to bring
about in his turn from the practice of science to the practice of writing
novels.

In 2001, in an interview in *The Minnesota Review*, Jeffrey Williams
asked Powers: "what made you turn from science to literature?" Powers responded by explaining that as a child he "took huge amounts of
pleasure in being able to solve problems in very different intellectual
disciplines," and that he thought he would become "one sort of scientist
or another." He grew frustrated, however, with the increasing specialization in the sciences. Later, doing a master's degree in literature, he also
became frustrated with the increasing specialization in literary criticism.
He told Williams that he "wanted to arrive somewhere where [he] could
be the last generalist and do that in good faith." It was only through writing novels that Powers thought he could "preserve that sense of multiplicity, of generalism."

I want to consider, therefore, how a novel about cancer (or at least
Richard Powers' novel about cancer), rather than other forms of writing about cancer, including medical case histories, scientific studies, and
even first-person illness narratives, might be particularly suited to reveal
the complexity of cancer, and even inspire or invent new approaches to

understanding the relationship between health and human rights. Powers' turning from science to literature is not, in the end, a turning away from science. He turns from the practice of doing science to the practice of literature and then turns his literature to science in the hopes of preserving a sense of multiplicity and generalness, not simply for literature, but for science too.[5] This is a question of method as much as form. It is not simply that literature can help us understand how science is done because it presents "real" portraits of science and scientists. Rather, what interests me is the possibility that literature might provide a new approach to doing science. The fact that this notion seems somewhat absurd indicates the current asymmetrical relation between the practices of science and literature with regards to method; surely literature has nothing to contribute to the hallowed scientific method. However, this is precisely what Susan Squier (2004) argued in her recent book, *Liminal Lives*. Squier approached "both literature and science as technologies" that have the potential to bring new objects into being (p. 3). She called for an interdisciplinary methodology that would put literature and science in conversation. "Because of its particular epistemological positioning between knowledge and unawareness," Squier believes, "literature is able to hold open a zone of exploration that other mediations (political, social, scientific, and economic) foreclose. Literature thus offers an alternative to the expert discourse that…has become socially and epistemologically dominant" (p. 22).

HEALTH AND THE EMERGENCY OF THE LONG TERM

In "Toward an Ethics of the Future," Jérôme Bindé (2000), director of the Analysis and Forecasting Office of UNESCO, discussed the relationship modern societies have to time. According to Bindé (2000), "modern societies suffer from a distorted relationship to time" because they are preoccupied with the present (p. 51). To correct this preoccupation, Bindé believes we must shift our attention from that which might bring gains in the immediate term towards an ethic that attempts to take account of the future. Bindé is concerned then with the temporality of human rights, or more precisely, with how we exercise human rights temporally. Bindé reminded us that

> [o]ur relation to time has enormous economic, social, political, and ecological consequences. All over the world, the citizens of today are claiming rights over citizens of tomorrow, threatening their well-being and at times their lives, and we are beginning to realize that we are jeopardizing the exercise by future generations of their human rights. (p. 51)

The failure to take account of the human rights of future generations often gets rationalized by the citizens of today, through what Bindé (2000) called a "logic of emergency," which shuts down our capacity to think beyond our present moment (p. 52). He is aware that one way in which a logic of emergency in the present threatens the human rights of countless future generations is with policies that favor short-term economic development over and against those that support long-term environmental sustainability. What we need to counter this logic of emergency, Bindé (2000) maintained, is a "new paradoxical form of emergency, the emergency of the long term" (p. 56). This requires us to recognize our responsibilities not just to those closest to us in time and space, but to others, across space and time (Bindé, 2000, p. 59). Bindé's project is to rehabilitate the long term. I contend that Richard Powers has a similar project in *Gain*.

The story that *Gain* tells is a long one. It begins in the town of Lacewood in the last decade before the turn of the millennium. Despite its somewhat unremarkable position in middle America, from the outset, we learn that present-day Lacewood is connected via a long history to countless other events in the past, small and great, and to countless other places across the globe, near and far:

> Lacewood's trace began everywhere: London, Boston, Fiji, Disappointment Bay. But everywhere's trail ended in this town, where folks made things. Some mornings, when the sun shone, history vanished. The long road of arrival disappeared, lost in the journey still in store. (Powers, 1998, p. 3)

How can we make this vanished history reappear? How can we locate traces that begin everywhere? And how does this vanished history and the traces that connect us to it relate to our current situation, and to the health of individuals and entire communities in the present and future? Powers' ambition in *Gain* is to make the long road of arrival reappear in narrative, in order to reveal the connection between it and the journey still in store. By rehabilitating the long term in narrative, Powers, like Bindé, suggested that a new concept of time will bring into being "a new method of solving problems—namely, anticipation" (Bindé, 2000, pp. 55–56).

On the one hand, then, *Gain* is a historical novel, and the histories it presents are multiple and complex; on the other hand, and relatedly, it is a novel that hopes to anticipate a different future. *Gain* is the history of a town, Lacewood; the history of a corporation, Clare; the histories of two families, the Clares and the Bodeys; and the history of an individual with ovarian cancer, Laura Bodey. Woven into and across these multiple histories—of town, company, families, and individuals—are two other histories that I think of as intertwined metahistories: the history of capitalism and the history of cancer. What is the relationship between all of these histories? How might making their interrelatedness visible help us anticipate a future different from the present? Although his story is multilayered, Powers (1998) also suggested ways to unweave, at least in narrative, the strands that constitute the history of the present. "There must have been a time when Lacewood did not mean Clare, Incorporated," he wrote (p. 4). "But no one remembered it. No one alive was old enough to recall. The two names always came joined in the same breath" (p. 4). To unjoin the two names, Powers began his story long before this joining of Clare to Lacewood, indeed, long before Clare incorporated in order to show that this story—this present story of one woman's ovarian cancer—was never inevitable.

Modes of Ordering Ovarian-Cancer Causation

In *Organizing Modernity*, John Law (1994) offered what he calls a "modest sociology" that starts from the premise that "the social, all the social world, is complex and messy" (p. 5). Law is not interested in delineating *the* or even *a* modern social order, but in exploring modes, or practices of ordering in modernity. He wanted to investigate "ordering" as verb, not "order" as noun (p. 5). Human subjects are not the only agents who do the ordering, however. Law attempted to articulate a "relational materialism" that takes account of both human actors, and nonhuman and material actors. For Law, discourses and technologies "form a crucial part of any ordering" (p. 24).

I want to think about two different, though not unrelated, modes of ordering ovarian-cancer causation as presented in *Gain*: the genetic and the environmental, or a mode of ordering cancer causation from the inside out and a mode of ordering cancer causation from the outside in. In their essay, "The Health of Black Folk: Disease, Class, and Ideology in Science," originally published in 1986, Nancy Krieger and Mary Bassett (1993) also discussed what they call genetic and environmental models that help to explain the scientific "fact" that "black Americans are sicker and die younger than whites" (p. 161). They contended that neither the genetic nor environmental models, when utilized by either conservatives or liberals, can account for the effects of oppression on the health of African Americans. Krieger and Bassett argued that a Marxist and antiracist model of disease causation offers more effective strategies for improving the health of African Americans (pp. 168–169). Their analysis is an important early critique of the neoliberalization of health care policy. My own analysis diverges from theirs in that my understanding of the environmental model as presented in *Gain* is influenced by the rhetoric and practices of environmental-justice activism, which problematizes the economic disparities that capitalism creates, and uncovers the effects of these disparities on the health of particular communities.

In presenting their Marxist and antiracist counter-model, Krieger and Bassett (1993) are critical of a liberal view that "fetishizes the environment" (p. 165). In this view

> individuals are harmed by inanimate objects, physical forces, or unfortunate social conditions (like poverty)—by *things* rather than by people. That these objects or social circumstances are *creations* of society is hidden by the veil of "natural science." Consequently,

the "environment" is viewed as a natural and neutral category, defined as all that is external to individuals. What is not seen is the ways in which the underlying structure of racial oppression and class exploitation—which are relationships among people, not between people and things—shape the "environments" of the groups created by these relations. (pp. 165–166)

Although I agree with Krieger and Bassett's insistence on the need to understand and transform the underlying structures of oppression in order to improve health outcomes, I do not believe that such an analysis can proceed without accounting for people *and* things, and the relation between people and things. In the next section I will focus predominately on the human actors—doctors, patients, and their loved ones—doing the ordering of ovarian cancer. However, as the section following will show, there are also nonhuman actors contributing to this ordering, including various discourses and technologies. In this case, there is the soap factory, its techniques of soap manufacture, and its organizational structure, as well as the Clare Corporation's many products and the way these products are packaged and marketed. These discourses and technologies are capitalist, of course, and they are articulated by, and benefit, particular people within the capitalist system, but they are not simply experienced as a relationship between people. In my understanding of complexity and cancer, things matter; indeed, they shape the way an individual experiences the world.

ASKING THE CAUSAL QUESTION

After surgery to remove her ovaries, Laura Bodey, a lifelong resident of Lacewood, tentatively asks her doctor about the cause of her cancer, a question she will reformulate several times over the course of the novel. She has difficulty finding the words. Indeed, even broaching the question seems to separate her questioning self from the self who has cancer:

> Laura hears herself speak, from inside a shortwave radio set. "What is the cause?" She cannot say *of ovarian cancer*. She cannot say *of this*. "Is it genetic?"

She just wants to know how much of this is her fault. Whether she should have done something. Might still do something. Whether she would have had to go through this even if she lived better. Whether Ellen. (Powers, 1998, p. 76)

Laura's initial inquiry into the cause of her ovarian cancer connects her illness to both the past and future: Is it genetic? Can it be traced to past generations of her family? Is her daughter Ellen at increased risk for this disease in the future because of Ellen's genetic connection to her? Laura wants to know the temporality of her illness, and, perhaps unsurprisingly, her first queries about the temporality of ovarian cancer *move from the inside out*: from her body to its immediate relations in the past, present, and future.

Dr. Jenkins, the surgeon, answers her question by admitting the question cannot be answered definitively: "'Sometimes.' The doctor frowns. 'Nobody really knows for certain'" (Powers, 1998, p. 76). Laura's ex-husband Don is exasperated by this answer that suggests both unknowingness and multiplicity. He wants definitive answers, and he wants them now: "'Which is it? *Sometimes*, or *Nobody knows?*'" (Powers, 1998, p. 76). Don wants the world and Laura's ovarian cancer properly ordered. He wants and expects the doctor to be able to simplify Laura's cancer; he does not want the doctor to make it complex, or worse still, not to know how to order it for him (and for Laura, though what becomes apparent in the novel is that what Laura wants and needs is not always what Don thinks she should want or need).[6] Unlike Don, Laura wants to ask other questions about what we do not know about ovarian cancer: How could she have had this dreaded disease without knowing? How long does she have to live? These other questions are also about the time of her cancer: When did it begin and when will it end—or, in literary terms, what is its narrative arc? However, Laura does not ask these questions about the time of her cancer because "the words [*"How long do I have to live?"*] seem rude" within the institutional spaces of medicine, and she doesn't want to "embarrass the physician that way" (Powers, 1998, p. 76). Laura seems to recognize intuitively that medicine does not have answers to the question of the time of illness, and to even ask such questions of medicine is an affront to what medicine is and what it can do.

When Laura later discusses chemotherapeutic treatments with her oncologist, she asks again about cause at the end of the interview, when the specialist asks her, "'Is there anything else we can help you with?'" (Powers, 1998, p. 99). Again, she is uncertain how to formulate the question, or even if she wants to formulate it. She asks, "'What causes... why do I have this?'" (p. 99). Her oncologist responds by reassuring her that her question is completely "natural," though at the same time unanswerable:

> "Now, that's a very natural question. Almost everyone who comes into this office wants to know the answer to that one." He grins, indulging her understandable human frailty. "I wish I knew the answer. Ovarian cancer does follow at least three distinct hereditary patterns."
>
> "No one I'm related to has ever been near it." (Powers, 1998, p. 99)

Laura's response is somewhat odd as she connects the hereditary with the spatial and environmental: no one she is related to has been near it, suggesting that the notion of proximity presented here combines the genetic and the spatial. In Laura's speculative mode of ordering her own ovarian cancer, nearness to someone genetically also suggests spatial or environmental nearness. The oncologist responds to Laura's distancing of her own situation from the hereditary mode of ordering by shrugging again. According to Powers, the specialist's shrugging "gesture falls on his shoulders like a favorite windbreaker," as he admits, "'There's also some evidence that provoking agents, either combined with or inducing an alteration in the immune system...'" (Powers, 1998, p. 99). Laura is unable to pay attention to the rest of his evasive nonanswer masquerading as an answer. Powers ends this sentence with an ellipsis suggesting that in this scene the two cannot communicate across the "phrase regimens" that separate them, and signaling, in the terminology of Jean-Francois Lyotard, a différend[7] that opens up between Laura's question about cause and the doctor's answer. The "natural" question can only be answered if the cause can be attributed to "nature," that is, nature in the sense of "distinct hereditary patterns." Beyond that, the evidence is sketchy, and therefore offered only as a shrugging gesture meant to deflect further questions. Laura Bodey does not yet know the questions she needs to ask, and the doctor does not want or know how to anticipate them.

During her 6 months of chemotherapy, the treatment, more than the disease itself, transforms Laura's world, again from the inside out. Her body becomes her whole world, not through her increased knowledge of it, but paradoxically, from her surprising lack of knowledge of it. The narrator explained how:

> No one really knows their real body. Hers has turned electric, buzzed, frizzy. Her internal organs go some horrid shade of Naugahyde. No one knows what food really smells like. Well-being is nothing but an imposter, a beautiful girl who turns into a hag at neap tide when the spell breaks and reason at last sees through her (Powers, 1998, p. 114).

Laura's life is reduced to the internal spaces of her body and the temporality of cancer treatments: "A day dripped out in microseconds outlasts the idea of time" (Powers, 1998, p. 113). A body undergoing such treatments does not remember how it once felt before the treatments, nor does it anticipate feeling, in the future, other than how it feels now. Memory and anticipation—projection of time into the past and future—are lost to Laura and her transformed body as "the calendar shrinks to its barest rituals" (Powers, p. 19), recalling Bindé's "logic of emergency" at the level of the individual body.

Recovering from her treatments, Laura Bodey's world begins to widen beyond the spaces of her own body when her daughter Ellen shows her an article from the local newspaper: "EPA LISTS LOCAL EMISSIONS. Annual Toxic Release Inventory Details Area's Plants" (Powers, 1998, p. 139). Laura peruses the article, but cannot connect the newspaper story to her particular situation. "'Here,' Ellen says. 'Ri-ight here'" (p. 139). In this gesture, which is a counter-gesture to the oncologist's earlier shrugging off of Laura's questions, Ellen tries to focus her mother's attention outside of herself, to the newspaper story, and the possibility of a relationship between her cancer and her environment. Ellen's "Here. Ri-ight here" brings the story about the toxic emissions into their town and home in an attempt to make her mother consider the question about the relationship of these toxins to her cancer. Ellen's gesture also empha- sizes that in fact the toxins may already be here, now, and that they may have been here for some time. The article ranks Illinois counties by toxic discharge. "Lacewood, Sawgak, Vermilion, Champaign, Iroquois. Area's top carcinogenic chemical environs. Benzene, formaldehyde, dichlorodi- fluoromethane, epichlorohydin…" (Powers, p. 139). Laura, who has wor- ried that, genetically, she may be the cause of her daughter's future cancer, is offered an alternative mode of ordering the cause of her cancer by her daughter: not caused from the inside out "naturally," but rather from the outside in, "unnaturally." Laura is still not ready to hear this possibility, and in an attempt to comfort her daughter, repeats the two phrases that contain her doctor's deferral of questions of cause and responsibility— "they don't know what causes ovarian" and "probably genetic" (Powers, p. 139)—though, of course, neither phrase is much comfort to Ellen.

Only when an outsider comes into Laura Bodey's home and relates Bodey's experience of cancer to the experience of others in the commu- nity does the possibility that something in the environment has caused her cancer begin to sink in. Laura invites her visitor, a black woman named Janine, into her home, and immediately the stranger recognizes how Laura is suffering. It is unclear whether Janine is a Jehovah's Wit- ness or a cancer activist engaged in a house-by-house mapping project of her community, but she is clearly meant to suggest both the spiritual and the political aspects of witnessing.

> "Your skin getting thin? Hurt to touch? You bruise easily? All
> your hair scram at once? Ringing in your ears?"
>   Laura nods. It feels good. This stranger has asked her more
> questions in three minutes than her doctor has in three months.
> (Powers, 1998, pp. 188–189)

Janine's questions are not asked simply to elicit information, they are asked as a practice of witnessing to another person's suffering. Laura learns that Janine's husband died of cancer, and that he worked at Clare, and that Janine believes working at Clare caused his cancer. When Laura expresses surprise at Janine's certainty about cause and effect, Janine responds,

> "You gotta start reading the papers, honey."
> "I know. I do. I mean my daughter showed me…"
> The cup wavers at Janine's lips. "That EPA story? That's old news. Where was the EPA twenty years ago? Thirty years ago? No. Everybody waits until the last minute. Then it's 'Okay, who didn't wipe their shoes?'" (Powers, 1998, p. 189)

Though she only makes a brief appearance in this story, Janine is an important figure in Powers' narrative. She comes into Laura's home as witness to her community and its long history of disease. By caring for her dying husband and by canvassing her community, Janine has seen the effects of environmental toxins. She also understands the temporal aspects of witnessing; she knows that to suggest that the crisis has suddenly come upon this town and its people is to forget that the time of disease is much longer than the time of any one individual's illness.

Moreover, she recognizes that the question of what constitutes evidence of environmental illness is complex. The evidence—the traces of toxins in the home—will not be discovered by looking at individual behavior in the present ("who didn't wipe their shoes?"), but by looking back at a history that has vanished. Only by rehabilitating the long term historically might we recognize the emergency of the long term in the present moment and anticipate a different future. Powers also argued that countering a disease that has possibly come from the outside in cannot mean closing our doors to the community around us. As Bindé demonstrated, we must let others in, in order to make connections beyond ourselves and to move beyond such private acts as remembering to wipe our feet before entering someone's home.

When Laura next sees her doctor, she "asks point-blank": "'Dr. Archer. Can cancer have environmental causes?'" (Powers, 1998, p. 191). He objects to her loose framing of her question, first telling her, smugly, cancer "is not cancer, is not cancer," and then asking her to define environmental (p. 191). Although this is an awkward moment between doctor and patient, it demonstrates that the experiences of cancer are multiple, as do the other conversations between doctors and patient presented in *Gain*. The doctor contributes to this as much as Laura does. Or, perhaps it is more accurate to say that Powers reveals in the différend between them that cancer can never be the same thing for Dr. Archer as it is for Laura Bodey. By repeating how cancer is not cancer, is not cancer, the doctor emphasizes that cancer is not one thing, and wants Laura to clarify which particular cancer she is asking about. This seems willfully obtuse or even arrogant of him. After all, what other cancer would a patient with ovarian cancer be asking about? At the same time, Powers hints here that there might be something to gain from thinking about cancer more generally—by compounding our approach to cancer and its causes, rather than simplifying it.

Laura is undaunted by Dr. Archer's defensive posture, and she continues to press him by clarifying her original question: "Can it come from something you eat or drink? Some kind of exposure?" (Powers, 1998, p. 191). Dr. Archer reaches, "slowly, as if he's very tired," for a binder above his desk, which the narrator described as, "clearly the answer file of last resort" (p. 191). He reads to Laura from an NIH consensus paper that noted that the cause of ovarian cancer is unknown, but that some women are at a higher risk for developing the disease. In the consensus Dr. Archer presents, there is no mention of possible environmental causes. Still, Laura pushes him, asking, if there can be outbreaks of ovarian cancer, to which he responds, "[w]e don't see much if any clustering of ovarian" cases (p. 192). Almost despite himself, however, he does offer some additional information: "Immigrants to this country do show higher incidence rates after living here about twenty years" (p. 192). Still hopeful for something other than the genetic mode of ordering ovarian cancer causation, Laura speculates, "That would sort of suggest an environmental reason, no?" (p. 192). Dr. Archer gestures to the NIH file, as if everything there is to know and say about the experience and event of ovarian cancer is contained in that file (even while it explicitly stated that there is still much we do not know). We are not privy to Dr. Archer's reason for bringing up immigrants, but in this figure our understanding of environment gets multiplied across time and space. Movement across space matters, but so does the passing of time, complicating the question of what changes for immigrants between then and now, between that place and this place.

What is problematic about this scene is that scientific knowledge becomes the end of the conversation not the beginning. Dr. Archer uses it to trump other knowledges when he tells Laura, "There is no evidence of ovarian cancer being caused by anything you might read about in the newspaper" (Powers, 1998, p. 192). Her questions about cause are no longer "natural," they are now an irritant, a waste of time. What is missing from Dr. Archer's practice of medicine is not simply an empathic relationship with his patient, but an understanding of the different temporalities of disease, illness, and medicine, and an ability to place Laura Bodey's questions, the newspaper articles about EPA reports of cancer hot spots, and the NIH consensus report in a much longer history of practices of medicine and scientific consensus. To trace this history is to begin to anticipate future practices and other consensuses. In its presentation of multiple modes of ordering ovarian-cancer causation, *Gain* does not simplistically render either the genetic or the environmental mode as the "answer file of last resort." Powers suggests instead that ovarian cancer is complex and messy. Indeed, the genetic cannot be separated neatly from the environmental. Again, the question remains open as to what changes for immigrants and their families. One thing is certain: we will not find the answer or answers to this causation conundrum by assuming that we already know all we need to know, or do not need to know, about ovarian cancer.

MAKING SOAP, MAKING THE CANCER-INDUSTRIAL COMPLEX

In his attempt to present the temporal complexity of ovarian cancer, Powers juxtaposes the long history of a capitalist enterprise—soap making—with the history of both a particular town where this making happens and the people who do the making.[8] Laura Bodey's relatively short personal history gets told along with—indeed, interwoven among—these longer histories. In doing so, Powers demonstrated the constitutive, not incidental, relationship between Laura Bodey's life and death from cancer, and the much longer histories and larger spaces of capitalism. Just as the time of cancer stretches beyond Laura's particular illness and medicine's treatment of it, the spaces of cancer are expanded beyond her body and the medical spaces of her treatment to her home and its connection to the Clare Corporation and the wider world. *Gain* gives form to the "Cancer-Industrial Complex." It makes links between an industry and an illness, between a form of making and a form of unmaking.

In her much-circulated essay "Welcome to Cancerland" first published in *Harper's* in 2001, Barbara Ehrenreich defined the "Cancer Industrial Complex" as "the multinational corporate enterprise that with the one hand doles out carcinogens and disease and, with the other, offers expensive, semi-toxic pharmaceutical treatments" (p. 52). Ehrenreich's piece is a diatribe against what she calls mainstream "breast-cancer culture," in which women are infantilized and made to believe that the only proper response to a breast cancer diagnosis is for the person with cancer and her loved ones to become consumers of "the cornucopia of pink-ribboned-themed breast-cancer products" (Ehrenreich, 2001, p. 46). More importantly, however, the essay is a general critique of what Ehrenreich (2001) saw as the wholly privatized response to breast cancer, signaled by an emphasis on consumption and "relentless brightsiding," that is, the ideology of maintaining a positive attitude at all costs as one faces the challenges of breast cancer (p. 49).

What is missing in this normative response, according to Ehrenreich, is anger, and a feminist political analysis that asks why so many women suffer from this disease and why treatments, often more than the disease itself, are the cause of so much suffering. What can we do to prevent cancer in the first place? How can we improve treatments such that they are not more awful to endure than the cancer itself (Ehrenreich, 2001, p. 49)? "In the harshest judgment," Ehrenreich (2001) asserted, "the breast-cancer cult serves as an accomplice in global poisoning—normalizing cancer, prettying it up, even presenting it, perversely, as a positive and enviable experience" (p. 53). I do not refer to Ehrenreich's argument in some detail here because the experience and event of ovarian cancer is the same as the experience and event of breast cancer. "Cancer," we recall, "is not cancer, is not cancer." This is so not just biologically but socially and culturally as well. Rather, what is interesting is that Ehrenreich uses the essay form to effectively present the Cancer-Industrial Complex. Likewise, Powers uses the novel form to present an image of the structure of the Cancer-Industrial Complex. Through his genealogy of the Clare family and its soap-making factory, which eventually becomes the Clare Corporation, Powers represents not only the present effects of the Cancer-Industrial Complex, but also its historical emergence. He shows the long history of soap production, from its production in the home to its production in a factory, from soap as household craft to soap as market commodity.

Two charts in *Gain* help demonstrate this complex visually. The first presents a plan for "chemical recirculation" in the Clare family's soap-making factory that, we are told, was developed in the late 19th century by James Neeland, who, for his innovations, was placed in "charge of one of the country's first industrial labs" (Powers, 1998, p. 170). Powers (1998) described chemical recirculation as the dream of the chemist: "turning the refuse from every transmuting process back into the supply path of another" (p. 170). We learn that Neeland has been influenced by developments at alkali factories in England, where

> chemists rolled a giant hoop around a regenerating hub, a wheel outputting its own inputs, its rim spinning off target substances, each the potential feed for whole new industries, each new industry a feed for the next. Neeland made a chart of the great wheel and hung it upon his laboratory wall, for all his assistants to study. (p. 170)

Neeland's chart may represent the dream of the chemist, but it doesn't tell the whole story of the process of soap making, even schematically. Although the chart appears to be a representation of a complete and closed system, in reality

Neeland's chart failed to include every substance that the process produced. Decades of live experiment upon British alkali towns now showed...[this] process to be cruelly inefficient. For every unit of sulfur that created wealth, two units rained back down upon wealth's beneficiaries as crippling soot and sulfurous drizzle. (Powers, 1998, p. 172)

What is gained in this "live experiment?" Powers gives us an image of civilization and its underside in the transformation of these British alkali towns.[9] If we look, we can see with our own eyes the smoke in the towns' air and the black stains on the towns' architecture. But what of that which we cannot see, the leftovers from the process that seep into the groundwater and enter homes undetected? How will the people of the towns pay for this? How are we to "see" the transformation of their bodies and genetic material? How do we chart the gains and losses across many generations?

The second chart in *Gain* that represents the Cancer-Industrial Complex shows the overall structure of operations at Clare Soap and Chemical in 1909. The goods produced by Clare Soap and Chemical are broken down into "personal goods" (including "tonics and salves," "alcoholic beverages," "lard and foodstuffs," and "soaps and candles") and "industrial goods" (including "bleaches," "anesthetics and disinfectants," "agricultural chemicals," and "process chemicals") (Powers, 1998, p. 274). Around this time, Clare also began to develop its sales division, which marketed much more than Clare's products. According to their mantra, Clare offered a "new style of life" (p. 276). In the graphic breakdown of Clare's organizational structure, we see all the aspects of the cancer-industrial complex that Ehrenreich delineated, the goods that cause cancer and the goods that treat cancer made by the same corporation. The chart also reveals the centrality of the ideology of consumer citizenship: that our most meaningful sense of belonging comes from the essentially private act of consumption of personal goods, rather than from the public act of political participation.

These interconnections are also made in Powers' narrative. When Laura is getting an infusion of Taxol, Dr. Archer visits her on his rounds. "Thank God for the home team, huh?" he says. Fuzzy from the drugs and confused by his comment, Laura can only respond by repeating "Home...?" Dr. Archer crows enthusiastically, "The home team! Our local gravy train." Laura is still confused, and only begins to understand when Dr. Archer clarifies for her, in the language of a good consumer citizen, "Stuff's brought to you by the same folks who took the fat out of deep-fat frying." Finally, what Dr. Archer is getting at hits home; the drug is made at "home." "Clare makes this?" Laura ventures, and Dr. Archer explained that it's slightly more complicated than that: "No. That would be Bristol-Myers Squibb. NoDoz, Ban, and a few cancer and AIDS gold mines. But Clare sells them cheap materials" (Powers, 1998, p. 151). Personal goods, industrial goods, and a new style of life: they're all on the chart, built into the structure of the company.

PRACTICES OF WITNESSING OVARIAN CANCER

Gain challenges the notion that the best response to cancer is in the creation of a "new style of life," where the cancer survivor always looks on the bright side of his or her experience. Just as it presents multiple temporalities and spaces of cancer, *Gain* also presents multiple practices of witnessing the disease. In her provocative essay on the representation of environmental toxins and the perception of risk in *Gain* and in Don Delillo's *White Noise* (1986), Ursula Heise (2004) argued that *Gain* presents an underlying capitalist system that cannot be changed or even effectively challenged. "Against the complex system of Clare's global body," she contends, "the local bodies of individuals or small communities are powerless" (Heise, 2004, p. 376). I disagree with Heise's pessimistic diagnosis of the essential impotence of individual and collective agency described in *Gain*, because it fails to consider the multiplicity of practices of witnessing, as well as the novel's temporal challenge to the logic of emergency. If we believe that we must transform the "complex system of Clare's global body" in the present moment, then we are bound to fail. By rehabilitating the long term, we see how efforts that begin now may not produce effects for years to come. Moreover, by bringing into being an emergency of the long term, we free the imaginations of individuals and small communities to make connections with others beyond their particular time and place.

I want to conclude by discussing the multiple practices of witnessing that *Gain* describes. Powers does not really suggest that one practice of witnessing is better than another. Instead, his goal is to demonstrate that the transformation of these global structures will be as complex as their emergence has been. There are four domains that I want to focus on here: suffering, the law, radical politics, and science. I have already described in some detail Laura Bodey's slow coming to consciousness about the possibility of an environmental mode of ordering ovarian-cancer causation, and it should be apparent from that discussion that Laura Bodey is an essentially passive figure in Powers' narrative. Her first reaction to her cancer is to believe it is somehow her own fault, and she is later reluctant to join a class action against the Clare Corporation that charges it with releasing toxins into the environment. Several commentators on *Gain*, including Heise, noted that Bodey's name is meant to suggest the word "body" (Heise, 2004; Scott, 1998; Williams, 1999).[10] Heise also points out the connections Powers makes between the "incorporated" company, its legal form of personhood, and Bodey's corporeality. In an interview, Powers has explained that "[t]he book is a dialogue between two individuals: the real individual, the forty-two year-old woman, dying of ovarian cancer, and the Clare corporation, which under the law of the land is an individual, enjoying due process" (Williams, 1999).[11] It is clear that these two protagonists are in many ways stereotypically gendered: Laura as passive female, and the Clare Corporation as active male. However, I contend that Laura Bodey's passivity might be read as a radical form of passivity, in the sense that it represents her willingness to withstand suffering without also heroicizing the experience of suffering and her identity as a sufferer. Bodey is not a "bright-sider." Nor does she ever become, even for a moment, a cancer survivor. What she does become is more and more ill, even as she tries to remain engaged in her children's lives. Eventually, inevitably, she dies of ovarian cancer. Hers is not a good or noble death; it is ordinary. Even so, the loss cannot be calculated.

Calculating loss is what the class action attempts to do, albeit crudely. Laura resists Don's attempts to make her participate in the lawsuit, telling him, "It's just not something...cancer's not something that I really want to profit from" (Powers, 1998, p. 285). However, Don argues that this sort of attitude allows the company to profit while "everybody else picks up the tab" (p. 285). For Don, the law can determine who has gained and who has lost, and this possibility of calculating loss and gain in monetary terms is crucial to his mode of ordering the world. In his view, the courts offer a space and practice of witnessing that can account for loss. This is enough for him, though not for Laura. She tells him, "A court is not going to tell me what I need to know" (p. 287).

Heise (2004) saw Don as the one character in the novel who, in his "[i]ndefatigable...search for accurate and comprehensive information," manages to achieve "some measure of knowledge and success in the struggle with Clare" (pp. 375–376). Although I find Don a compelling character, I read his approach to Laura's cancer and the possible connection to toxins produced by Clare as just one of several practices of witnessing that are, in combination and over the long term, potentially effective. Don has faith that through his own research practices he can obtain enough knowledge, and that this knowledge can be brought before the law, where justice can be achieved. Is this naïve? Not necessarily. Just as Powers presents Laura's radical passivity as one practice of witnessing cancer, he also suggests Don's knowledge gathering and use of the courts as another. We might think of this as a liberal practice of witnessing cancer, and Powers seems to want us to see it as one tactic in a larger nexus of responses.

In *From the Ground Up*, Luke W. Cole and Sheila R. Foster (2000) analyzed the tactics and strategies of the environmental justice movement. They noted that the law is one domain in which environmental justice is often sought, but they argued that it may not be the most effective one. Cole and Foster wrote,

Tactically, taking environmental problems out of the streets and into the courts has proven, in many instances, to be a mistake. In struggles between private industry and a host community, there are two types of power: the power of money and the power of people. Private industry has the money, while communities have people; this disparity in resources is evident in many environmental justice cases...In court, industry has access to the best lawyers, scientists, and government officials money can buy; to have a chance, a community group must often hire expensive experts. Relying on lawyers, rather than on a community's own actions, necessarily involves having just one or two people speaking for the community. On the other hand, a community-based political organizing strategy can be broad and participatory and can include all members of the community. (pp. 129–30)

Along with Janine's brief visit with Laura Bodey, we get one other glimpse of what might be considered a "community-based political organizing strategy" in *Gain*. As Laura lies dying, she is heavily medicated with morphine, but is still able to watch the news. Powers (1998) told us "she watches the local news, the state news, the national news, the international. Trawling. Something still out there, something she mustn't miss" (p. 342). Powers hinted that what she mustn't miss isn't the resolution of the Clare class action, which "drags on" (p. 342). When she does finally catch a glimpse of that something still out there that she mustn't miss, she thinks she dreams what she sees: "Through the morphine, Laura dreams that her own daughter crashes the local news cameras. Strange fantasy, where kids from the local high school take to the streets. Then Ellen is there at bedside, thrilled, telling her it was real" (Powers, 1998, p. 342). Powers gave us a dream-like image of the potential of radical politics; the "strange fantasy" of the people confronting power might actually become a reality.

In *Gain* we are presented with multiple forms of struggle, multiple practices of witnessing: Laura's radical passivity, Don's attempts to become an expert and to use the law, Ellen's direct-action politics, and finally (and it is the final image in *Gain*), science as a practice of witnessing. The science that Powers has in mind doesn't yet exist; it is a future science that must still be imagined. We learn that Laura and Don's son Tim, the youngest member of the Bodey family, has become a computer scientist, who

> hooked up with an interdisciplinary research group working on a computing solution to the protein folding problem. They sought to write a program—a whole library, in fact—that would take an amino acid sequence and predict exactly how it would fold up. For if they could find the folded enzyme's shape, they would know how the molecule behaved. And knowledge of enzyme behavior was the key to a cell's life and death. (Powers, 1998, p. 355)

The interdisciplinary team sought to create a method "to make anything [a] damaged cell called out for" (p. 355). This "universal chemical assembly plant" will produce cures, and the narrator tells us, "no one needed to name the first cure that would roll off their production line" (p. 355). We are perhaps back to a genetic mode of ordering ovarian-cancer causation, but it is not disconnected from the nonscientific fact of a young boy's loss of his mother to cancer. While this loss cannot be adequately calculated, Powers suggests it can be witnessed by a science motivated by such loss. Tim invests "his lump-sum buy-off" from the class action into this interdisciplinary scientific enterprise (p. 354). "The sum had been compounding forever, waiting for a chance to revenge its earning. The figure was now huge, a considerable bankroll. And softly, Tim suggested that it might be time for the little group of them to incorporate" (p. 355). Surprisingly, perhaps, *Gain* ends with the practice of incorporation, but I read this incorporation not, or not only, in the specific sense of "the document creating or legalizing a corporation," but more generally, as "the action of incorporating two or more things, or one thing *with* (*in, into...*) another."[12] As Powers has shown us, the moment of incorporation—of bringing together multiple stories and practices—is the result of a long history that connects, in this case, a supposedly objective scientific enterprise to one family's very subjective experience of loss. On the molecular level, we have to find a very specific method to unfold the protein, but this practice will never tell us all we need to know about the experience and event of ovarian cancer. For that, we must compound our interest.

References

Barsamian, D. (2000). *The checkbook and the cruise missile: Conversations with Arundhati Roy*. Cambridge, MA: South End Press.

Bindé, J. (2000). Toward an ethics of the future. *Public Culture, 12*(1), 51–72.

Cole, L., & Foster, S. (2000). *From the ground up: Environmental racism and the rise of the environmental justice movement*. New York: New York University Press.

Delillo, D. (1986). *White noise*. New York: Penguin.

Diedrich, L. (2004). "Without us all told": Paul Monette's vigilant witnessing to the AIDS crisis. *Literature and Medicine, 23*(1), 112–127.

Diedrich, L. (2005). A bioethics of failure: Anti-heroic cancer narratives. In M. Shildrick & R. Mykitiuk (Eds.), *Ethics of the body: Postconventional challenges* (pp. 135–152). Cumberland, RI: The MIT Press.

Diedrich, L. (2007). *Treatments: Negotiating bodies, language and politics in illness narratives*, Minneapolis, MN: University of Minnesota Press.

Diedrich, L. (2008). Visions of politics, time, and nation: Arundhati Roy's challenge to the experts. In V. Hesford & L. Diedrich (Eds.), *Feminist time against nation time* (pp. 131–148). Lanham, MD: Lexington Books.

Donadio, R. (2005, August 7). Truth is stronger than fiction. *New York Times Book Review*, p. 27.

Ehrenrich, E. (2001, November). Welcome to Cancerland: A mammogram leads to a cult of pink kitsch. *Harper's*, 43–53.

Heise, U. (2004). Toxins, drugs, and global systems: Risk and narrative in the contemporary novel. In P. Freese & C. Harris (Eds.), *Science, technology, and the humanities in recent American fiction* (pp. 343–381). Essen, Germany: Die Blaue Eule. (Originally published in *American Literature, 74*, 747–778.)

Krieger, N., and Bassett, M. (1993). The health of black folk: Disease, class, and ideology in science. In S. Harding (Ed.), *The "racial" economy of science: Toward a democratic future* (pp. 161–169). Indianapolis, IN: University of Indiana Press. (Originally published in *Monthly Review*, July–August, 1986.)

Law, J. (1994). *Organizing Modernity*. Oxford: Blackwell.

Law, J., & Mol, A. (2002). Complexities: An introduction. In J. Law & A. Mol (Eds.), *Complexities: Social studies of knowledge practices* (p. 1). Durham, NC: Duke University Press.

Lyotard, J.-F. (1998). *The differend: Phrases in dispute* (G. Van Den Abbeele, Trans.). Minneapolis, MN: University of Minnesota Press.

McClintock, A. (1995) *Imperial leather*. New York and London: Routledge.

Miller, L. (1998, July 23). The Salon interview—Richard Powers. *Salon.* Retrieved March 6, 2008, from http://www.salon.com/books/int/1998/07/cov_si_23inta.html

Mol, A. (2002). *The body multiple: Ontology in medical practice*. Durham, NC: Duke University Press.

Oliver, K. (2001). *Witnessing: Beyond recognition*. Minneapolis, MN: University of Minnesota Press.

Powers, R. (1996). *Prisoner's Dilemma*. New York: HarperCollins.

Powers, R. (1998). *Gain*. New York: Picador.

Powers, R. (2001). *Plowing the dark*. New York: Picador.

Roy, A. (1999). *The cost of living*. New York: The Modern Library.

Scott, A. (1998). A matter of life and death. *New York Review of Books, 45*(20), 38–42.

Squier, S. (2004). *Liminal lives: Imagining the human at the frontiers of biomedicine.* Durham, NC: Duke University Press.

Williams, J. (2001). The last generalist: An interview with Richard Powers. *Minnesota Review*, 52–53. Retrieved March 3, 2008, from http://www.theminnesotareview.org/journal/ns52/powers.htm

ENDNOTES

1. My use of the terms "compound" and "simple" is meant to suggest forms of capital accumulation. In *Gain*, Powers wants us to consider how technological advances create interest not only on the principle, but on the interest as well. He implies that the calculation of what we have gained with technology is not a simple matter; we have to learn to do the math better if we are to properly calculate change over time and across space.

2. Already I am reducing the complexity of each of these temporal and spatial domains by presenting them, for the sake of my analysis, as singular and discrete.

3. For further discussion of Oliver's philosophical work on witnessing in relation to Paul Monette's autobiographical writings about AIDS, see my essay, "Without Us All Told" (Diedrich, 2004).

4. Roy's frequent use of capitalization, as in, for example, "Big Dams," is meant to highlight how certain things obtain mythic status and are therefore perceived as beyond question. For an analysis of what I call Roy's "metaphysics and epistemology of small things that she believes must oppose the supremacy of Big Things," see my essay, "Visions of Politics, Time, and Nation: Arundhati Roy's Challenge to the Experts" (Diedrich, 2008).

5. Likewise, Roy turns her novelist's skill to understand the issues of Big Dams and nuclear proliferation. In an interview she described her approach:

> I started reading. I went to the valley, I met the activists, and felt that the movement needed to tell its story in a way which is accessible to an ordinary reader. It needed a novelist's skill. It's a complex issue, and much of the time the establishment depends on the fact that people don't understand. I wanted to build a narrative that could puncture that—to deal with all their arguments, to deal with their facts and figures, to counter them in a way ordinary people could understand. (Barsamian, 2004, p. 102)

6. Part of what is appealing about this portrait of a former marriage is that it shows how the relationship between Don and Laura continues to be negotiated through the event of Laura's ovarian cancer. The reader gets a sense both of why their marriage did not last, and why something else between them has lasted.

7. Throughout his work, Lyotard (1998) identified an infinite number of phrase regimens, which are various "mode[s] of presenting a universe" that are incommensurate and not translatable from one mode to the next (p. 128). Despite this fundamental incommensurability, Lyotard understands that the failure to link phrase regimens might lead not to paralysis or further suffering (though it certainly might), but to a lot of "searching…to find new rules for forming and linking phrases that are able to express the differend disclosed by the feeling" (p. 13). The hyphen that separates the two subject positions in the phrase "doctor-patient relationship" signals a différend. What happens when both sides begin searching for new rules for forming and linking phrases between these subject positions? I further explore this question and the searching it engenders in my essay, "A Bioethics of Failure: Anti-Heroic Cancer Narratives" (Diedrich, 2005) and Treatments: Negotiating Bodies, Language, and Politics in Illness Narratives (Diedrich 2007) (especially the conclusion, "Towards an Ethics of Failure").

8. The factory, broadly conceived, is an important space in Powers' work. For example, in *Prisoner's Dilemma* (1996), he investigated the history of the Disney Corporation as an image factory, and in *Plowing the Dark* (2001), he investigated a high-tech company that makes virtual reality. In all of his work, Powers analysed the complicated structures of making that bring into being new objects, images, realities, and even new forms of being.

9. In "Soft-Soaping Empire: Commodity Racism and Imperial Advertising," a chapter in her 1995 book *Imperial Leather*, Anne McClintock looked at the relationship between "soap and civilization" (p. 207). McClintock (1995) told a "soap saga," which goes like this:

> At the beginning of the nineteenth century, soap was a scarce and humdrum item and washing a cursory activity at best. A few decades later, the manufacture of soap had burgeoned into an imperial commerce; Victorian cleaning rituals were peddled globally as the God-given sign of Britain's evolutionary superiority, and soap was invested with magical, fetish powers. (p. 207)

According to McClintock (1995), because soap "purportedly belongs in the female realm of domesticity, soap is figured as beyond history and beyond politics proper" (p. 209). In her work, she begins to tell a social history of soap, one which emphasizes the "fetish ritual" of cleanliness (p. 211). Powers' novel might be said to offer a literary supplement to McClintock's psychoanalytic approach.

10. According to Heise (2004), the point of juxtaposing the two narrative strands…is to show how the corporate body and the individual body depend

on each other, and how the corporate organism can become a lethal threat to the individual one. More than any single substance and more even than the whole array of products it delivers, it is the corporation as a social form that kills Laura Bodey. (p. 372)

11. See also Laura Miller (1998).
12. These definitions were taken from the Oxford English Dictionary, retrieved September 10, 2006, from http://dictionary.oed.com.

CHAPTER 5

UNEXPECTED SIDE EFFECTS:

UNCOVERING LOCAL IMPACTS
OF KNOWLEDGE PROLIFERATION
ABOUT HIV METABOLIC DISORDER
IN TWO DISTINCT POPULATIONS

Cindy Patton

I finally went and decided to bone up on it myself and find out really what I was in store for and stuff…[I found out] mostly about the disease—and then I talked to my doctor about treatment and she never got into the particulars about what I would be in store for—she basically told me don't worry about it—like you don't even need to go there so let's not even you know worry or ask yourself about it…I ended up finding out more and more because the nurses were coming over to see [my partner] so they'd talk to me and tell me everything. So I ended up finding out a lot through them because of [partner's] meds and stuff.

—Interview with 36-year-old white female involved in
HIV support community among drug users (2004)

* * * * *

MD: What is your understanding of why you are here?

The patient reports his viral load and CD4 count and informs the doctor that he started protease inhibitors [PIs] six months prior. "I'm a poster boy for PIs!" He says. However, he has experienced a great increase in his triglycerides, which he and his HIV physician believe has resulted from taking the protease inhibitor, Ritonavir®. MD reviews his cholesterol counts. "These are new numbers for me," the patient says, contrasting his facility with viral load and CD4 measures against his knowledge of HDL, LDL, and triglyceride values—"I'm not used to these numbers." He informs MD that he attended a public talk given by the doctor the previous week. "I listened with great interest," he says, pulling out the power point slide copy with his notes.

—Fields Notes (2003); from observation of the intake interview of a 43-year-old white gay male at a specialized HIV lipids clinic

During 2003 and 2004, I conducted a pilot study in Vancouver, British Columbia, of HIV-positive people's understanding of the emergent side effects that are now known as HIV metabolic disorder.[1] Combining clinical ethnography, interviews with patients and patient advocates, and observation of public-education activities hosted by a local treatment-information project, I sought to understand what—and through what channels—individuals came to know about and experience this complex of side effects.[2] I was particularly interested in differences in levels of knowledge, and even more in the styles of making sense of that knowledge. Conventional knowledge attitudes behaviors practices (KABP) studies of HIV knowledge have long been used to demonstrate "levels" of knowledge and are based on standardized questions (often with adjustments for cultural differences). This type of survey, conducted in virtually every corner of the globe, has shown high levels of awareness of, and intention to engage in, "safe practices" in diverse study populations.

I might have conducted such a survey to document levels of knowledge of this "new" information on HIV metabolic disorder and to establish the "intention to change" diet, drug regimen, and physical activity, as per prescriptions of physicians and nutritionists. However, as I will make clear in this chapter, the information that was being rapidly disseminated during the period of the pilot was still equivocal—not a very "clean" environment in which to ascertain who knew what about HIV metabolic disorder.[3] For a variety of obvious reasons then, I rejected the much-criticized KABP approach, but I also designed my project differently for a less obvious reason: although I was interested in the uptake and use of a "new" category of HIV-related knowledge among men and women of different social classes (as were my funders), I was equally interested in the reflexive relationship between groups of people in different information-giving, information-receiving, and information-exchanging cultures loosely linked via (1) their consumption of mass media and (2) their participation in the HIV care system. I did not intend to exclude the classic markers that are used to analyze the so-called social determinants of health (here, social class and sex/gender), but rather wanted to raise questions about how these dimensions interrelate. Thus, I approached each "group"[4] in my study as a potential cultural unit, defined as much by neighborhood as by sex/gender, and as much by participation in social groupings and consumption of subcultural media as by "exposure" to mass media or access to Internet. By studying each group in a way that matched their interrelationship with the new knowledge, I was able to make some sense of the explicit differences in "level of knowledge" and style of interpretation and, I hope, to uncover the implications of these differences in the broader context of a medical system that struggles to treat patients on a very unequal playing field equally.

As indicated in the two quotes that opened this chapter, at the time of my study, and in this particular local context, gay men knew far more than poor women about HIV metabolic disorder. This would have been a frank finding of a KABP study, had I conducted one, and was useful information for the local treatment activism group, who soon conducted information sessions on side effects, treatment protocols, and so on, for women in the poor Vancouver neighborhood called the Downtown Eastside (DTES), where the first woman quoted in this chapter lived. The issue of why there were such differences is complex and relates to factors for which a KABP survey would have been a rather blunt instrument. Gay men and poor women are distributed in different, though adjacent neighborhoods (but importantly are both concentrated in neighborhoods), and while they use HIV services at the same hospital, their use of services is dramatically different, and the allied health- and community-support networks each group uses do not overlap much.

Because the dominance of KAPB surveys has so infiltrated even our popular thinking about how groups of people differ in relation to information/knowledge sources, there is a tendency, even in analyzing qualitative data, to reduce difference to flat variables. Thus, I reserve extensive analysis of my field notes and interviews for another essay, and instead consider here what conceptual framework might be required to understand the genesis of social differences in medical knowledge. This essay consists of two brief genealogies: firstly of the body said to be at risk of HIV metabolic disorder, and secondly of the gendered construction of HIV/AIDS as it is reflected in service provision. In the first part, I examine how a particular image of the body with AIDS was initially constituted in national and international media in relation to existing racist, gendered, and less explicitly, class constructions. In the second part, I explore how the interrelation between health-advocacy work and the effects of race, gender, and class formed the basis of two different, locally situated interpretive communities, which each invited different readings of the lipodystrophic body—that is, the body with HIV metabolic disorder. Finally, I speculate on the extent to which the broad mediascape informs (1) part of the "common sense" underpinning health planners' decisions about who needs what kind of care, and (2), reciprocally, the dynamics of the communities' influences on their members' decisions about when and how to seek care and to advocate for change.

MULTIPLE BODIES, TWO EPIDEMICS, ONE VIRUS

Over the last decades, much intellectual labor in semiotics, cultural studies, and anthropology has sought to understand how we come to our bodily sensibilities, how we come to carry ourselves as we do, how we create the mental constructs—many of which torment us—that we now think of as body image. Work on "the body" may stand as the most significant and sustained contribution of cultural studies, with its feminism, its form of political economy, its attention to the everyday, and its intellectual mobility across academic disciplines that are otherwise disconnected.

Second-wave feminists argued convincingly that a significant element in our understanding of what we look like and our perception of whether we are healthy arises in relationship to media images. The complex of ideas we gloss as "distorted body image" arises from the sociocultural location—people we physically live among—and the placement of oneself in the landscape of media images that are supposed to represent us. Of course, we know that people do not imitate media images in any simple way. Yet, it still seems that women in particular, with gay men hot on their heels, agonize a lot about whether they fit the beauty norms presented in the mainstream (in the case of women) and subcultural (in the case of gay men) media. To complicate matters further, in the midst of a declared epidemic of obesity, the science of body shape is still equivocal about whether the shapes and proportions individuals aspire to, or seek to avoid, are actually healthy or unhealthy. Nevertheless, these decades of debate among feminists—about the cultural roots of anorexia, about the social opprobrium towards "fat"—are the foundation of the work on representations of bodies with HIV.

From the earliest days of mainstream media coverage of HIV/AIDS— even in the early 1980s when a blackout on the topic was more or less in effect—the bodies of people living with AIDS were represented as "wasting." There were two versions of this image. The first came in the form of "before and after" pictures of gay men—for example, the widely circulated pictures of Hollywood hunk Rock Hudson, diagnosed in 1984 with late-stage HIV disease. Indeed, the international onslaught of media coverage of Rock Hudson set the standard for covering the human-interest side of the epidemic, as the diptych of Rock before and Rock after was reproduced on the local scale, with lesser or only regionally known persons diagnosed with advanced AIDS.[5] In a little recognized bid against generalized homophobia, the "before" picture, often a graduation photo, suggested that the category of "boy next door" could include gay men, while the second picture, or the "after" shot, took back this momentary suggestsion that gay men could be healthy by asserting AIDS as a conse-quence of the "gay lifestyle." It is important to note the undecidability of this diptych; the question that vexed mainstream readers was whether the man in the first image was "already gay," and later, "already infected." The many "you can't tell by looking" campaigns—explicitly about HIV, but implicitly, also about gayness—referred back to the diptych.

The second version of the wasting image was "the African." Unlike the gay diptych, this was a single photo, often of a solitary individual, in which it was almost impossible to tell if the frail body was male or female, child or adult. These interchangeable Africans were usually placed in a village context, or else appeared as lonely black bodies against the white sheets of what were meant to be understood as patently inadequate hos-pitals. Importantly, despite the fact that from the beginning of epidemio-logic attention to AIDS half the cases in Zaire, Kenya, and Cameroon were women, this gaunt image did not rely on gender iconography for its message: if white, the frail body was gay, and signified sexual devi-ance; if black, the frail body required no gender or sexuality, and signi-fied the hopelessness and poverty of a vague media version of an entire continent called "Africa." It is critical to recognize that, from the outset, AIDS was, politically and morally, two different epidemics, linked by a virus and carrying two messages: on the one hand we were supposed to understand that homosexuality is dangerous, and on the other, we were asked to accept that those left behind by capitalism would never catch up. Notably, the images used to represent AIDS in "Africa" were already widely circulated: editors might easily have passed off "African famine" photos as "the ravage of AIDS" photos. This is not the case for the representation of gay men.

We might recall that until the AIDS epidemic achieved its status as media staple in the mid-to-late 1980s, lesbians and gay men were hardly represented in the mainstream media at all (although "people like that" were already coded through decades of tabloid and pulp fiction representations). Thus, as various commentators and scholars have pointed out, while there were some representations of gay men prior to the epidemic, it was as the victims and perpetrators of AIDS that the now-naturalized image of the Western, urban, *gay man* achieved international visibility. In the course of about two years, gay men went from near invisibility to being the embodied representation of a pandemic disease. This lightning-fast "mediagenicity" occurred in parallel to, but not as a result of, the actions of gay and lesbian media activists who worked to achieve "positive images" of lesbians and gay men. The reality that the epidemic would demand stories that could be populated by earnest lesbians and gay men serving their community (queer "points of light" in the neoconservative slouch towards dismantling the welfare state through increasing volunteerism and collective work by "communities"—though, ideally, faith communities over sexual ones) was a massive blow to a generation of gay liberationists who, like feminist of the 1970s, wanted to radicalize alternative relationships, not valorize monogamous, long-term companionship.

The rise and fall of a particular advertising campaign in the gay press from the early 1980s illustrates and complicates our understanding of the role of the politics of visibility in the early days of the epidemic. This minor drama occurred on the cusp of the moment when gay men were forced to give up any sense that they had a private semiotics—a gay vernacular or gay counter-public space—safe from the moral judgments of mainstream society. In 1983 an advertising campaign for the newly released hepatitis B vaccine appeared very briefly in the gay press. The vaccine had been in trials in San Francisco. At the time, few outside the gay community realized the extent of the hepatitis B epidemic in urban "gayborhoods," and few today realize that the early AIDS movement was importantly presaged by the sexual-health activism in the late 1970s surrounding hepatitis B.

The black and white image of a frail man recumbent in a hospital bed might have tested well just a year earlier, when it would likely have been seen as a dramatization of the seriousness of hepatitis B among gay men, and something to be read only by gay men. However, two things had changed, and they had done so extremely quickly. First, early AIDS coverage had linked gauntness and AIDS in the public imagination, as the "gay plague" eclipsed all other gay men's health issues. Secondly, and perhaps even more importantly, gay men now understood themselves to be under the civic microscope for the behaviors that might or might not be linked to escalating rates of HIV transmission. Increasingly sensitized to the effects of living in what Foucault called a "carceral society," gay men perceived the hepatitis B advertisement as a representation of gay men as a whole. Gay activists attacked the advertisement, comparing the image to right-wing literature of the day, in which the gaunt, presumably dying gay man had replaced the flamboyant drag queen in a Pride march as the symbol of the "dangers of homosexuality."

Where gay activists had once sought broader public representation, gay community-based AIDS activists now contested images both within and outside of the gay community. With a certain amount of fanfare in the gay press, the hepatitis B advertisements—the revenue upon which the smaller newspapers in those pre-desktop-publishing days depended heavily—were quickly pulled from circulation. The image of thinness (though not the quest to be unfat) was doubly encoded by the mid-1980s, in both the intracommunity sign of ill health and the public sign to which homophobic sentiment could be attached. In this case, a new community was born, formed by an indeterminate number of urban gay men banding together. Such community offered new possibilities for responding to AIDS and interpreting knowledge about it: strategies about representation could be debated there, and on the community's behalf, public health dollars could be sought in order to create images of gay male health.

REPRESENTING WOMEN

The early establishment of two forms of wasting AIDS bodies—one "First World," white, gay male, and one "Third World," ungendered, and black—had implications for the representation of women and HIV. Even though women were diagnosed with AIDS before a name was even chosen for the syndrome, they were considered an enigma until the late 1980s. Initially, described as "prostitutes" or "addicts," women with HIV appeared not as people but as vectors between men. Early newspaper representations that sought visually to link AIDS and women consisted largely of hazy, dark, long shots of sex workers congregating around cars. It was probably the 1989 case of New York socialite Ali Gertz[6] that offered the first opportunity for the media to introduce a third moral logic related to HIV infected bodies. For this, it drew on the wasting body image and related it to white, middle-class (necessarily heterosexual) women. They did not use the "before and after" format though: showing a frail and ailing Ali Gertz would have diminished the wholesomeness required by the Pollyannaish optimism that accompanied the prognosis of white women with HIV/AIDS, and would have undermined the implied suggestion that they could catch a fatal disease but not actually die from it. Nor did the media invoke sexual libertinism, even though it was fairly clear that Ali Gertz was no stranger to the posh club scene. Indeed, the media went to great lengths to separate Ali Gertz from the women they represented as trading sex for money (see, e.g., Lambert, 1989). Instead, using this opportunity to create a new image of the person with AIDS, the media employed the "before" half of a gay male diptych and lashed it to the "before" picture of Gertz. Faced now with images from two apparently hip, urban heterosexuals, we were encouraged to read the former as the newly invented stealthy bisexual and the latter as a dupe, a woman (like you, dear reader!) "who couldn't tell that her man had a man."

In a deeply ironic way, this new articulation of the perky, postfeminist, white woman who could not pick out a bisexual man, decreased, rather than increased the space in which women might identify themselves as potentially contracting or already having HIV. The Ali Gertz story told them there was no way that nice girls could possibly know whether her man was bisexual, or that she might have contracted HIV. Thus, as the visual rhetoric of AIDS in North America consolidated in the late 1980s and early 1990s, there was a surplus of wasting imagery for white gay men and a lack of representation of illness for women. When women's ailing bodies were visible, they represented something other than women's experience—a metaphor for poverty, the crisis of African underdevelopment, the risk of infection to infants, the hazards (to men) of sex work.

THE MIRACLE OF MODERN MEDICINE

The mediascape and health-advocacy initiatives of the 1980s had several consequences for health-promotion and health-information campaigns of the period, which in turn served as the backdrop for the new images and issues that emerged when the protease inhibitors became available, and eventually came to inform the current reception of knowledge about HIV metabolic disorder. In the 1980s, the image of the wasting "AIDS victim," coupled with the widespread perception that HIV disease was invariably fatal, had an incalculable effect on the body image of gay men, resulting in two major problems for gay-male-health promotion. Firstly, beauty norms in the larger gay culture focused on a "healthy" look that, if difficult for most to obtain (either because of incompatible body shapes or due to actual HIV sequelae), was nonetheless widely cited as the cause of depression and feelings of exclusion. Paradoxically, coming out of the 1970s "Twiggy" look, the new "healthy" look featured muscles, minimal body hair, and good skin. Classified advertisements in gay newspapers and magazines increasingly invoked health as a dating criterion, with "healthy" coded as HIV-negative.

But because there were no images of women with AIDS iconographically comparable to those of gay men, and because women are media subjects as individuals, not communities, women as a group were deprived of identificatory possibilities ("that looks like me!"), and hence discouraged from seeing themselves as potentially at risk of contracting HIV from their sexual partners. Except perhaps in urban sex-work circles, where women might be concerned that customers would avoid them if they were perceived to have AIDS, women generally were not affected by the media representations of women with AIDS that periodically appeared in a similar way to how gay men were affected by the host of media images of gay men with HIV. As sexual consumers, both women and gay men increasingly relied on personal strategies for deciding who might be "risky" and how long that risk should be tolerated. Almost since the beginning of the epidemic (and no doubt before that), surveys of condom use (and hence, risk logic) have shown a trend towards decreased condom use over the course of a relationship, a quotidian practice raised to the level of explicit strategy in educational campaigns like one in Australia called "Talk, Test, Test, Trust." Safe-sex educators were never able to convince sexual actors to simply adopt a universal strategy of condoms every time and instead had to grapple with providing people with the best information to help them make decisions in the context of individual, site- or scene-specific decision-making strategies. For gay men, there was a shifting subcultural perception of "what a person with AIDS looks like" and, in turn, shifting strategies to avoid looking like such a person. Until the advent of new treatments in the 1990s, the look gay men avoided was gaunt and frail.

The drug companies that launched the first round of highly active antiretroviral (ARV) therapies, or HAART, known colloquially as the "AIDS cocktail," were quite aware of the shifting semiotics of gay-male culture. The first direct-to-consumer (DTC) advertisements featured masculine men climbing mountains, riding bicycles, hiking, and sailing. In one way, there was great pleasure in consuming these advertisements, a certain sense of revenge in their suggestion that gay men might beat the pants off their straight brothers who had all the cards stacked in their favor. However, these images were also poignant because they held out false hope that people with HIV could finally return to unfettered active lives.

There were virtually no DTC advertisements aimed at women[7]—although it must be admitted, women were not likely to become a big market for the new drugs in the United States because of their lack of high income levels, health care coverage, or community base from which to disseminate information about the new treatments, compared to gay men. The advertisements that did include women were either of a pleasant heterosexual couple, or simply a photo gallery of the "many faces of AIDS," as in the various earlier human-interest stories that used this visual strategy to "put a face on AIDS" (Patton, 1996). Given the dispersal of women across various communities, and the perception that few women had AIDS, there were no media outlets for DTC advertising of HIV medications to women—certainly not the women's magazines, which, while they might warn about HIV, were not about to routinely hail their audience as being likely to have contracted it or needing HIV medications (this, in sharp contrast to advertisements for herpes medications in current issues of these same magazines). Helen Kang (2005) has elaborated the strategies used in direct-to-physician HIV-drug advertising campaigns, and she points out that there are different objectives and different campaigns aimed at marketing drugs to consumers and to prescribing physicians. Interestingly, she finds that these direct-to-physician advertisements feature women far more commonly than the direct-to-consumer campaigns for the same drugs at the same moment. Thus, the bulk of the representations of women in HIV medication advertisements are aimed at defining, for doctors, who their female HIV patients might be.

Unfortunately, despite saving countless lives, components of HAART proved to have many side effects, among which is a noticeable change in the distribution and utilization of body fat. Some data suggests that these dyslipidemias lead to increased risk of cardiac problems for people taking HAART (Henry et al., 1998). However, concurrent theoretical and applied work in endocrinology that has clarified how the body utilizes and distributes fats makes it much less clear that (1) HAART alone results in the apparent increased risk, and that (2) body shape changes correlate with the predictors of cardiac risk (Kotler, 2002; Kotler, Rosenbaum, Wang, & Pierson, 1999; Sekhar et al., 2002). Despite the medical uncertainty regarding the precise cause and means of modulating these effects, analysis of this pilot project's data (including analysis of consumer newsletters, clinical encounters, and consumer attendance of educational seminars by physicians) made clear that HIV-positive people undergoing HAART held very strong opinions about the changes in their body shape.

Not only do they experience psychological effects relative to their body image (unsightly "lumps and bumps"), but they also believe that these shape changes are associated with increased risk of heart attack. Very little research has explored HIV-positive patients' experience of side effects like lipodystrophy, and that which does is primarily psychological, focusing on loss of self-esteem, rejection by partners, renewed fear of discrimination as they now "look like" a person with HIV, and potential nonadherence to drug regimens in an effort to avoid side effects (see Collins, Wagner, & Walmsley, 2000; Heath, Singer, O'Shaughnessy, Montaner, & Hogg, 2002; Oette et al., 2002), rather than exploring the social and cultural contexts in which various groups experience side effects, or do not experience them, as such. Indeed, most of this work comes from surveys or interviews with individuals who have presented for care following a crisis about side effects.

GENDERING EFFECTS

The clinical observational data from this study suggests that while gay men seem to "feel" better and have laboratory results confirming the success of their drug regimes, they actually "looked worse" (Field Notes, 2003, n.p.). Indeed, as one gay man noted, "You used to think someone had AIDS if they were skinny, now you look for lumps in weird places" (Field Notes, 2003, n.p.). Folklore and scientific confirmation have identified several specific patterns of bodily change, some related to long-term HIV infection and some to components of the antiretroviral combination therapy. Because the fundamental mechanism of these changes is endocrinologic, there are differences in effects between men and women, and in how these effects are expressed. For example, men in general tend to accumulate fat in the belly, while women accumulate fat around the hips. The abdominal accumulation is highly accentuated for people on Crixivan, but the visual effect of this is far more noticeable in men, partly due to basic differences in body shape, and partly because of the prior cultural signification of the pot-bellied male body (that he has "let himself go"). Besides, medium-build women with a similar abdominal distension would likely be read as "pregnant." Both men and women experience swelling in the breasts. For women this may go unnoticed. For men, it creates something of a gender crisis. One gay male patient I observed complained of getting "breasts." He said to his doctor: "I don't know if this will make any sense to you" (Field Notes, 2003, n.p.). When the doctor explained that this was part of the fat redistribution of HIV metabolic syndrome, he noted to the patient that they should also assess him for breast cancer, to which the patient replied, "Breast cancer??? Guys can get that?" (Field Notes, 2003, n.p.). Other studies report that women describe discomfort and psychological distress from exaggerated swelling. I would suggest, however, that when women notice these changes, they experience and interpret them against a lifetime of experience with cyclical breast size and tenderness changes, and in a cultural milieu that currently valorizes large breasts.

Furthermore, because much public health campaigning in the past few years has linked fatness and heart risk, many gay men now—with equivocal evidence to support them—perceive their HIV-drug regimes to be placing them at higher risk for cardiac events. As one man put it, "I thought I would die of the virus. Now I'm afraid I'm going to have a heart attack" (Field Notes, 2003, n.p.). For a complex of reasons, this concern was virtually absent among the women we interviewed. Firstly, because disadvantaged women are likely to discover they are seropositive or enter treatment only after a serious illness, the majority of the women we interviewed had experienced severe weight loss before going on medications. If they experienced fat redistribution after going on HAART, this was either welcomed, or viewed as just another physical change to be coped with. They were more likely to sustain the association between wasting and HIV than to see their weight gain as a public sign of their serostatus. Secondly, women's risk of heart attack is under-acknowledged in North America. As Barbara Ehrenreich (1983) pointed out decades ago in *Hearts of Men*, having a heart attack is represented as being something that happens to men. Even though there are news reports every few years about the shocking discovery of rising rates of heart attacks in women ("more women die of heart attacks than breast cancer," such reports often state), the media continue to largely represent men in general coverage of cardiac issues. Finally, it is actually not at all clear why heart-attack rates among women in general are increasing, or whether these factors, and not HIV medications, are the cause of cardiac risk among seropositive women. Much like the debates about whether the aging of the HIV-positive gay male cohort, or the HIV medications themselves are the cause of increased cardiac risk among HIV-positive gay men, it is hard to sort out the causes of increased cardiac risk among seropositive women.

The overall increase in female cigarette smoking is as likely a culprit as rising female obesity, and disadvantaged women are more often smokers than their middle-class counterparts. Moreover, disadvantaged women rarely have the financial means or social context to maintain a good diet or to engage in systematic cardiovascular exercise, making it very difficult to disentangle the relative contribution of poverty, poor diet, lack of exercise, and HIV to cardiac risk. While I believe they were partly being ironic, several women-interviewees noted that they had been quite "heavy" but had come to a "normal" size as a result of this HIV-related disease. Indeed, needing to ensure that they did not lose too much weight was a new concept for most of our interview subjects. One woman was gleeful rather than alarmed that she could now eat as much as she wanted and never gain weight. In this somatic logic, it seems unlikely that the characteristic fat-redistribution patterns associated with HIV metabolic disorder would be noticed until it became quite pronounced. In an interesting sense, the lack of clear public and subcultural images of women wasting or becoming lumpy seems to have relieved women with AIDS of the burden experienced by gay men of disguising their physical changes.

WHAT WOMEN KNOW: GENDER DIFFERENCES IN CARE PROVISION AND ACTIVISM

As I stated from the outset, the foundation of my impressions about gay men's recognition and interpretation of HIV metabolic disorder, as opposed to that of impoverished women, is constructed from two rather different kinds of data: clinical observation of gay men and interviews with women. Although I did not plan for this difference (I also interviewed gay men and observed one woman in the clinic), the dramatic difference has as much to do with the gender structuration of HIV care and HIV activism as it does with bad research design on my part. While I spent a considerable amount of time at the clinic over the course of about 18 months, I saw only one of the 8 or so women who attended the clinic during that time period, and I saw her at both intake and follow-up. There were about 400 men attending the clinic at that time, of whom I saw about 90, and I saw dozen or so of these multiple times. There are other endocrinologists in Vancouver who see HIV patients, and a portion of men with HIV metabolic disorder go to those specialists. HIV doctors have competing treatment theories, and this means that their referral networks are also somewhat distinct. Moreover, concerns about women's health and HIV 20 years ago led to the development of a clinical group that specializes in HIV care for women, and this group has its own consulting endocrinologists and conducts its own research on HIV metabolic disorder. The women we interviewed were identified through another clinic, located in the poverty-stricken Downtown Eastside (DTES), which serves the bulk of the Aboriginal population in that neighborhood. Although some of the women we interviewed had gone to the women's clinic, they were all currently attending one of the clinics in their own neighborhood. A conventional comparative study of men and women would have required crafting a relationship among these several clinics, which have their own histories, practices, and mutual antagonisms.

What is important to this essay, as I frame an explanation of why poor women's and middle-class gay men's understandings of HIV metabolic disorder are so different, is the social and medical reasons that underlie the skewing of the population of people who have HIV as opposed to those who have HIV *and* experience treatment side effects. Firstly, HIV metabolic disorder, like the discovery of HIV itself, appears most decisively among those who have been monitoring their health, and, in the case of dramatic fat redistribution, among those who have long experience of being on antiretroviral regimes. Furthermore, since the distribution of HIV/AIDS ARVs is already socially overdetermined—that is, there is a perception that drug injectors and other marginal people cannot stick to the complex regimes—the cohort of those who are impacted by effects of long-term treatment is similarly overdetermined. The general consequence of this—the predominance of gay men, and, to a much lesser extent, white women in long-term ARV treatment cohorts—is exacerbated at the local level by the fact that, despite being disproportionately infected compared with all other subpopulations, active drug users and HIV-positive Aboriginal persons, particularly young women, are much less likely to be receiving treatment of any kind.

One other compounding factor is that ARV-treatment protocols have changed rapidly and radically, with a trend towards delaying treatment among middle-class patients, who are likely to be compliant. This means that today, a newly infected person will be started on ARVs much later than those who were infected 5 years ago. Long-term survivors were likely to have gone on ARVs under the "hit early, hit hard" theory of the late 1980s to late 1990s. These (mostly male) patients would have been on almost all the various kinds of ARV, at some point, and would have developed viral resistance, requiring them to go on yet different drugs and different combinations. Thus, a significant percentage of the cohort of men seen at the HIV metabolic disorders clinic are individuals who, were they diagnosed today, would have continued many, many years before being medicated with ARVs. The effect of being medicated with ARVs "too early" is difficult to study, and no one wants to deal with the moral ramifications of having damaged the bodies of an entire generation of gay men. However, the toll of taking highly toxic drugs unnecessarily may well be one of the important underlying factors in the generally poor cardiovascular and metabolic health of long-term survivors.

All of these factors, along with the similarity between the side effects and typical aging, make it extremely difficult for doctors to sort out which of the metabolic and cardiac problems result from specific ARVs, which result from long-term treatment, which result from aging, and which result from long-term infection with HIV itself. Several of these factors differ according to sex: if aging itself is a major factor, for example, then there are likely to be important sex differences, since women are much less likely to have received treatment in the "hit early, hit hard" era (it was some years before drugs were trialed on women, and much of the access to early classes of drugs depended on enrolling in a study). Moreover, poor women with HIV have among the highest mortality rates because they get no care at all. Thus, current evaluations of side effects in women must take into account the fact that the women likely will have gone on regimens "late" in their HIV process and will have worse underlying sexual, cardiac, and metabolic health.

It is vital to recall that much of the success of early gay-health organizing is a result of the influence of feminism and the women's-health movement of the 1970s. Like the women's-health movement, gay men tried to educate health care providers about the particular social issues faced by gay men, highlighting the ways in which homophobia diminished gay men's health. Also, the gay men's health movement promoted sexual health and renamed stigmatized sexual activities in much the same way that that the women's-health movement promoted the idea of the "well woman." Women's-health advocates argued that menstruation, pregnancy, birthing, and menopause were "normal" aspects of women's physical lives, and not pathological conditions to be subjected to medical scrutiny. Similarly, gay-male-health activists countered both moral and medical discourse when they insisted that anal sex was not contrary to nature, but only one of a wide range of sexual expressions, indeed, a sexual expression also engaged in by "normal heterosexuals." Women's-health advocates argued that clinical intervention into, and medicalization of, the aforementioned basic female body states were means of controlling women. Similarly, gay men argued that pathologizing sex cast gay men as ignorant of, unable to, or unwilling to use health precautions like condoms, resulting in the transmission of sexually transmitted diseases that either destroyed their health or placed them directly under the control of public health policing.

Unfortunately, as has been widely documented, while the women's-health movement was very influential for the early gay men's health movement, and especially the HIV/AIDS movement, the women's-health movement somehow failed to quickly incorporate HIV/AIDS into the purview of women's-health activism. It took nearly a decade before the movement in North America as a whole recognized the significance of HIV/AIDS for women's health (feminists in developing countries, and indeed, feminists in the antipoverty movement, faced HIV much earlier than the mainstream women's-health movement). There are a number of reasons for this, but two stand out: Firstly, the women's-health movement of the 1970s had been organized around self-help, depathologizing women's bodies, and viewing women as essentially healthy. The early cases of AIDS in women were very dramatic; these women were, like the gay men lying next to them in hospitals, *very* sick, consumed by a frightening disease that, in the early years, seemed to epitomize the absolute opposite of the "well woman." While there were important early female activists in the PWA movement, they did not come from feminism, even if they did battle the sexism within the Persons With AIDS (PWA) movement and in the framing of HIV. In fact, despite the work of many individual feminists within the AIDS movement, it was not until the late 1980s and early 1990s, with the highly theatrical and vocal women's caucus of ACT UP, that feminism was visibly present in AIDS organizing. This involvement, however, was promoted by third-wave feminists who had little or no connection to the women's-health movement.

Secondly, the kinds of women who were reported early on as having contracted HIV were precisely the women whose lives and place in society had vexed not only second-wave feminists, but also first-wave feminists. These were poor women, black women, prostitutes, drug users, race and class traitors, renegades, and women on the margins of society. In a very important sense, their poverty, color, vocation, pleasures, and self-understandings stood in the way of their articulation as sisters, and instead made them into a kind of degendered "Other." This was not the women's-health movement's finest hour. However, eventually, through feminist practitioners working within and through rural women's centers and urban clinics, and through the important activities of ACT UP, the movement did form a very strong and activist network that continues to care and advocate for women with HIV/AIDS.

Although the National Association of People With AIDS (NAPWA) created an explicit inclusion mandate for women early on, recruiting and promoting women to its leadership positions, there were massive differences between gay men (and their communities) and women (in their multiple locations and networks). Thus, while gay men's health advocates were actively contesting the kinds of images that emerged around their bodies and their lives in the epidemic, women living with HIV/AIDS were largely abandoned by feminism because media-related activism in the women's movement was focused on promoting images of "well women," or fighting pornography and sexually explicit advertising. Drawing on the strategies and modest accomplishment of gay-media activists to get lesbians and gay men represented on their own terms, PWAs, especially men, had access to mainstream reporters, and had an independent media in which to circulate "good" information and develop a collective critique of mainstream media cover. The durability of individual, local gay communities that, by the mid-1980s, were mobilizing to cope with HIV/AIDS, and their interconnection to a larger national and even global "gay community," enabled a certain (though, many now complain, inaccurate) folk history and characteristic style of "reading" the media.

Women living with HIV/AIDS were neither members of the militating gay community, nor did they have a discursive lever to push for reconsideration of the women's-health movements' "well woman," antipathologizing discourse (cancer and psychiatric disorders were other problems for the "well woman" image). The various locales in which women were contracting and living with HIV/AIDS were less dynamically interconnected than those of gay men were. Their points of interpretive continuity and development of a critical attitude existed mostly in relation to mainstream media and in small, ephemeral support groups, or through their local HIV/AIDS-service organizations, the majority of which had some form of women's program early on. The problem experienced by women living with HIV/AIDS was not only the indirect pathologizing of their reproductive capacity. Rather, their essential (and probably in many respects ongoing) problem was that health care providers still failed to recognize that their patients might have HIV—a reality that is only exacerbated by the fact that women are located not in easily targeted, researchable communities, but in dispersed, multiple spaces.

If women live or work in a space that is identified as "risky" (sex-work venues, drug-trade venues, dilapidated neighborhoods which are often themselves economically tied to both organized and unorganized sex and drug trading), they are all too likely to be tested, and if positive, persuaded, or at least encouraged to start treatment. If this is not the case, however, that is, if they are white and middle class or living in a rural area or in a country outside of North America or Europe, then their symptoms are likely to be misdiagnosed or belatedly diagnosed. To a great extent, the situation of women in the urban developed world has dramatically improved: women are now diagnosed more effectively than they previously were, allowed to access treatments once denied to them because they were toxic to potential fetuses, and receiving many more services tailored to their specific health needs. However, if one adds poverty, homelessness, color, drug use, or sex trade to the situation, then barriers to accessing care and remaining in treatment become a significant problem for many women.

DIFFERENT INTERPRETATIONS, DIFFERENT SOCIAL EFFECTS

In this essay, I have tried to interrelate the changing representation of the gendered, raced, and classed person living with AIDS with the differential provision of care (for good and ill) of middle-class gay men and impoverished women, with attention paid to the small space for activism by women with HIV/AIDS, and to the activism by women in relation to the pandemic. This parallel genealogy provides some guidelines for interpreting what gay men and poor women have to say—in the clinic or in an interview—about their recognition, experience, and mitigation of HIV's symptoms and the side effects of drugs. In future analyses I will deal more directly with the discursive practices of the two groups. Here, I want to offer a few practical suggestions for health care and service providers and activists.

Firstly, while fat redistribution seems less often to be troublesome for women, the prevalence among them of type II diabetes and the changes in cardiac risk should be of great concern, since these are two areas where women in general are already poorly served, not least because both diabetes and cardiac risk are also known to have biological and social differences according to sex/gender. The important differences create a challenge for feminist AIDS activists who have, for 2 decades, asked researchers—primarily virologic researchers developing treatments—to be gender blind in their drug trials by not excluding women. In the case of HIV metabolic disorder, we are in a different scientific universe, and one in which complex factors like hormonal differences between men and women, the use of birth control pills, and differences in sugar metabolism processes may, in fact, make for important sex-related differences in diagnosis and treatment outcomes. Moreover, the long-recognized cofactors of stress, diet, exercise, and smoking are socially distributed with marked gender and class differences. As I have suggested, these affect patterns and modalities of health promotion and care.

Although the current problem of metabolic side effects does not seem to weigh as heavily on poor women as on middle-class gay men, the reasons for this are no cause for celebration. Fewer women receive medications, and many women lead chaotic and stressful lives in which side effects like fat redistribution, if noticed at all, are not a top priority on a long list of worries. Given its roots in the two-part image of the wasting body, the public AIDS discourse still provides very little space for women to articulate their experience of HIV treatment. The organizational and cultural successes of gay communities do not translate for women because women do not form a tidy subculture in which they might develop alternative norms and systems of information exchange.

The logic of women's-health advocacy itself remains problematic, since it must sometimes ask the medical systems to be sex blind and, at other times, press them to focus on sex and gender. Finally, the different kinds of science that come into play in treating people with HIV also fail to recognize women's biological differences from men, or they highlight these at inappropriate times. Although much has changed in the overall picture of AIDS treatment in North America, there is still relatively little attention paid to how new treatments are working out for women, and when, and whether to add side-effect-mitigating treatments to the pill burden of people who have little support for maintaining treatment and self-care regimens.

One of my original research questions concerned this last issue. My funders understood the question thusly: Do metabolic side effects cause people to become noncompliant with their ARVs? The style of analysis I offer here suggests a reframing of that question, and my data also provides a partial answer. Given that individual people inhabit their social locations in different ways (there is a complex mix of different labels whose relative importance shifts by context and over time), it may not make sense at all to aggregate individual treatment histories into something like social determinations of adherence. The broad patterns are very interesting to note, and may have relevance for the siting of services and supports for people who want to undergo treatment. What is helpful to understand, it seems to me, is the imaginative context in which people come to have bodily experience labeled as a "side effect," and it is this that I have preliminarily attempted to describe here. However, it is also valuable to understand the space in which treatments are deployed; that is, we need to understand the ebb and flow of care provision—which, in the case of HIV, is intimately tied to advocacy and activism. AIDS activism (part so-called empowerment of people living with HIV/AIDS, part assault on the mediascape in which HIV is represented) also sets the framework for interpreting new information about HIV. The highly local experience of noticing a lump or bump is interconnected with global science through the border-free dispersion of clinical information about HIV metabolic disorder, but only when the clinician and the activist who give a name to that experience recognize that the woman in front of them may actually be expressing a part of the new complex of symptoms.

REFERENCES

Bourdieu, P. (1977). *Outline of a theory of practice* (R. Nice, Trans.). Cambridge: Cambridge University Press.

Collins, E., Wagner, C., & Walmsley, S. (2000). Psychosocial impact of the lipodystrophy syndrome in HIV infection. *AIDS Read, 10*(9), 546–551.

Ehrenreich, B. (1983). *The hearts of men: American dreams and the flight from commitment.* New York: Anchor Books/Doubleday.

Field notes. (2003). From the Understanding Lipids Project, gathered by Patton, C. Unpublished.

Field notes. (2006). From the Accidental Communities Project, gathered by C. Patton & J. Liesch. Unpublished.

Heath, K., Singer, J., O'Shaughnessy, M., Montaner, J., & Hogg, R. (2002) Intentional nonadherence due to adverse symptoms associated with anti-retroviral therapy. *Journal of Acquired Immune Deficiency Syndromes, 31*(2), 211–217.

Henry, K., Melroe, H., Huebsch, J., Hermundson, J., Levine, C., Swensen, L., et al. (1998). Severe premature coronary artery disease with protease inhibitors. *The Lancet, 351*(9112), 1328.

Interview with HIV-positive female. (2004). Vancouver: Understanding Lipids Project.

Kang, H. (2005). *Queer bricolage: A visual study of HIV prescription drug advertising.* Unpublished master's thesis, University of Toronto.

Kotler, D., Rosenbaum, K., Wang, J., & Pierson, R. (1990). Studies of body composition and fat distribution in HIV-infected and control subjects. *Journal of Acquired Immune Deficiency Syndromes and Human Retrovirology, 20*(3), 228–237.

Kotler, D. (2002). *Update on lipodystrophy...or is it just lipoatrophy?* Review of papers from the XIV International AIDS Conference, Barcelona. Available from Medscape. Retrieved March 3, 2008, from http://www.medscape.com/viewarticle/439480?src=search

Lambert, B. (1989, March 11). Unlikely AIDS sufferer's message: Even you can get AIDS. *New York Times.* Retrieved March 3, 2008, from http://query.nytimes.com/gst/fullpage.html?res=950DE7D71639F932 A25750C0A96F948260&sec=&spon=&pagewanted=all

Oette, M., Juretzko, P., Kroidl, A., Sagir, A., Wettstein, M., Siegrist, J., et al. (2002). Lipodystrophy syndrome and self-assessment of well-being and physical appearance in HIV-positive patients. *AIDS Patient Care and STDs, 16*(9), 413–417.

Patton, C. 1996. *Fatal advice.* Durham, NC: Duke University Press.

Sekhar, R., Jahoor, F., White, A., Pownall, H., Visnegarwala, F., Rodriguez-Barradas, M., et al. (2002). Metabolic basis of HIV-lipodystrophy syndrome. *American Journal of Physiology—Endocrinology and Metabolism, 283*(2), E332–E337.

ENDNOTES

1. These side effects include: increase in low density lipoprotein (LDL) and decrease in high density lipoprotein (HDL); spiking triglycerides; an incremental trend towards Type II diabetes; development of fatty deposits on the back of the neck, abdomen, and breasts; dramatic thinning of face, forearms, and calves. The condition of individuals with abnormal cholesterol and blood-sugar values worsens, and cardiovascular events, especially heart attacks, appear to increase among those on certain HIV medications, especially smokers.

2. The clinic in which I worked was a new service at the hospital that has provided, since the early 1980s, the bulk of the more technical HIV services available in Vancouver (originally HIV testing for the virus and a dedicated ward—later, clinical trials and a multidisciplinary treatment unit). The treatment-information group has been active in the city since the early 1990s, and several more came into being during the 18 months of my study. While they hosted several public forums on HIV metabolic disorder, these were mainly attended by gay men, and a few male IV drug users active in the Vancouver Persons With AIDS (PWA) organization.

   Midway through my pilot, a treatment-information series was held specifically for women, hosted at a clinic in the downtown Eastside (DTES), where the majority of the impoverished HIV-positive women in Vancouver live. As is often found in studies of information "uptake," the structure of information flow was ragged in this series because the structure of groups processing information was ragged.

   The interviews with poor women that I draw on here predate this series of educational events and provide a good picture of the knowledge about HIV metabolic disorder (and side effects more generally) in a cultural space into which much HIV information arrives and is processed. Although the interviews are less revealing with regards to the exact routes through which information flows, we can make some provisional guesses about the interpretative community constituted by this loosely connected group of HIV-positive women.

3. Like "AIDS," initially called "gay cancer," "gay bowel syndrome," and "gay-related immune deficiency," the side-effects of HIV medication have undergone renaming. Initially, gay men themselves raised the question of whether

certain changes in their bodies might be caused by the drugs—hence, names like "Crix-belly" for the abdominal thickening believed to be associated with Crixivan. Once the apparent increase in heart attacks was noticed, clinics began to establish HIV lipids and cardiovascular clinics. However, the fact that men who were experiencing these problems were older, were smokers in disproportionately high numbers (who is going to tell a dying person to quit smoking?), and had generally had HIV for more than 10 years, confounded studies designed to pinpoint the cause of these changes. By the end of 2004, the name "HIV metabolic disorders" came into vogue to cover the range of problems related to both long-term infection with HIV and the various medications that exerted a direct effect on clinical measures (especially triglycerides) and body shape.

4. The "groups" were provisionally defined as doctors, treatment advocates, attendees of the lipids clinic, and economically disadvantaged drug users. These groups have different ontological statuses in relation to one another and are asymmetrical, a design problem only if groups are intended to be "comparable"; that is, only if I want to measure some attribute like level of knowledge. Instead, I was interested in the "habitus" of each group. Habitus, French sociologist, Pierre Bourdieu's (1977) notion of an acquired system of generative cognitive, behavioral, perceptual schemes "objectively adjusted to the particular conditions in which it is constituted" (p. 95), applies equally well to residents of a neighborhood as to inhabitants of a professional identity.

5. It is useful to recall here the history of the AIDS diagnosis. It was 1985 when a virus—eventually named Human Immunodeficiency Virus, or HIV—was identified and definitively associated with the wide complex of symptoms, most of which are diseases in themselves, that was thereafter called AIDS. The duration of asymptomatic infection was unknown in those early days, as was the question of whether all HIV infections led to the full course of illness and death (this was not established until the late 1980s). Thus, in the crucial period during which the image of the person living with AIDS (PWA) was established, the vast majority of those known to have HIV had already developed AIDS. Indeed, until the late 1980s, most people sought testing only after they developed symptoms they believed might be related to HIV infection. These early images were not only pre-"AIDS cocktail" (ironically, the drugs associated with pronounced lipodystrophy), but, as I will elaborate in this essay, of a product of the time when those noticed by medicine and the media were already sick.

6. This section condenses my longer analysis of the Gertz case, which appears as a chapter in *Last Served? Gendering the HIV Pandemic* (Patton, 1994).

7. There is one very curious advertisement that features a heavily muscled woman throwing a javelin. It is hard to read the advertisement as depicting an HIV-positive woman. Rather, she seems to represent something strong that can hit the mark.

CHAPTER 6

WOMEN, VIOLENCE, AND MENTAL ILLNESS:

AN EVOLVING FEMINIST CRITIQUE

Marina Morrow

[I]sn't there a danger that they [subjugated knowledges] will be recoded, recolonized by these unitary discourses which, having first disqualified them and having ignored them when they reappeared, may now be ready to reannex them and include them in their own discourses and their own power-knowledge effects?

—Foucault (2003, p. 11)

In this chapter, I will explore what happens when the medical/psychological frameworks that discursively produce what we call "mental illness" are challenged by feminists and those allied with antipsychiatry and psychiatric-survivor movements, all of whom offer different explanations for the host of experiences of women in distress, particularly as that distress correlates with experiences of violence.[1] I highlight the tensions between the discourses of biopsychiatry and more sociopolitical framings of the causes of mental illness[2] through a review of feminists' historical attempts to get women's interconnected experiences of violence[3] and mental distress recognized by psychiatry, and through an examination of the contemporary development by feminists of "trauma informed" and "trauma specific" services[4] for use in the mental health and substance use fields. I draw on Canadian examples to illustrate the challenges and potential benefits of feminists working more closely with mental health professionals, which has occurred in this country in recent years, and which has impacted the kinds of critiques being brought to bear on psychiatry. Concurrent neoliberal state reforms, with their attendant effects on Canadian women's organizations, are the backdrop against which this investigation must take place, and I note these effects on feminist critiques throughout. I conclude the chapter with a cautious endorsement of current feminist efforts to influence mental-health care practices while taking care to heed Burstow's (2005) criticism of the feminist movement for failing to ally itself closely enough with psychiatric-survivor movements that are the source of the "subjugated knowledges" powering feminist attempts at institutional change.

In my efforts to understand approaches to women's mental health as shaped by broader structural and institutional forces, I have been influenced by a growing body of feminist and poststructuralist analyses that view the nexus of power and knowledge as a central element of social relations. In particular, Foucault's genealogical methodology is relevant to my argument. Here, I put his genealogy to work, in order to produce a critical analysis that maps the evolving influence of psychiatric medicine on definitions affecting the labeling, treatment, and experience of women who are considered "mad" (Corker & Shakespeare, 2002). Specifically, I build on Foucault's notion that a deeper understanding of the official "scientific" discourses of, in this instance, psychiatry, placed alongside the "insurrectionary" knowledge derived from local and experiential knowledge, can be useful for devising strategies for change. As Foucault (2003) noted, "we can give the name "genealogy" to this coupling together of scholarly erudition and local memories, which allows us to constitute a historical knowledge of struggles and to make use of that knowledge in contemporary tactics" (p. 8).

Diedrich (2007) has similarly drawn on Foucault, arguing that his notion of "an antiscience born from struggle" is useful in both disability studies and the disability rights movement in that it facilitates a challenge to expert scientific knowledge sets (Foucault, 2003, p. 9). I would extend this analysis to suggest that "antisciences" are comparably useful in the study of mental illness when applied to "desubjugate historical knowledges" and "reactivate local knowledges" (Foucault, 2003, p. 10). Genealogies also have the potential to identify how various forms of knowledge are transformed through their interaction with dominant discourses, and to track what gets lost in the translation from "subjugated" to "official" knowledge.

Central to my analysis is Foucault's suggestion that the behavior of individuals and groups is pervasively controlled through standards of "normality," which are disseminated by a range of normative knowledges such as criminology, medicine, psychology, and psychiatry, and that individuals become invested in these categories and classifications such that they become the agents of their own normalization (Dreyfus & Rabinow, 1982). Thus, since social control is achieved not through direct forms of repression, but through scientific and administrative discourses, it follows that these discourses should be the subject of interrogation. For this reason, feminists are drawn to Foucault's genealogical method; here is a way of exploring how women's experiences and self-understandings are constructed in and by the power relations that they now seek to transform (Diamond & Quinby, 1988). The focus on discourse allows the tracing of a "kind of large-scale conversation in and through texts" that tells us multiple stories about historical struggles (Devault & McCoy, 2002, p. 772).

PSYCHIATRIC INSTITUTIONALIZATION AND "TRAUMA-INFORMED" CARE: AN EXAMPLE

In a 1998 study conducted at Riverview Psychiatric Hospital, outside Vancouver, British Columbia (RVH),[5] inpatients (women and men) were surveyed regarding their experiences of violence and abuse (Fisher,

1998). The results showed that 58% of the women had been physically and/or sexually abused as children and confirmed other Canadian and U.S. findings that women mental health inpatient populations experience higher rates of violence and sexual exploitation than the general population does (Craine, Henson, & Colliver, 1988; Firsten, 1991; Fisher, 1998; Muenzenmaier, Mayer, & Struening, 1993). The study was conducted with the sanction of the provincial government of the time, and a key feminist bureaucrat worked to give it a high profile, with the aim of securing funding for staff training that would improve the care of survivors of violence. However, the release of the findings prompted resistance from the RVH administration, who upheld the argument from the psychiatrists working at RVH that encouraging discussions about violence amongst such a "vulnerable" and "ill" population would be detrimental and run counter to good psychiatric practice. The prevailing belief was that psychiatrists work with mental illness, not histories of violence, which are seen as secondary and unrelated to the person's current "symptomology." For example, psychiatrists at RVH indicated that if they thought their patients had experienced violence they would refer them to supports in the community upon discharge—in other words, such a history would be dealt with elsewhere and by others. After the release of Fisher's (1998) findings, attempts to discuss increasing the staff's capacity, and that of members of the profession of psychiatry to work with survivors of violence went nowhere.

A year later, in an attempt to return these concerns to prominence (and to find a way to account for the government money originally given to RVH to develop violence-related programming), the original government bureaucrat contracted a women's-health-research organization (the British Columbia Centre of Excellence for Women's Health) to conduct a study exploring the mental-health care system's response to women-survivors of violence. The political strategy was to increase the research evidence on a problem—the mutually determining relationship between violence and mental health—that was already known to many working in the field of mental health who did not, however, have the means or political influence to demand increased training in order to help them work with survivors of violence. As the principal investigator on this study, I operated within a feminist critical-psychology framework, generating an analysis that showed how the biomedical focus of the mental health system actively worked against recognizing violence in the lives of women with mental illness (Morrow, 2002). Furthermore, our research found that some women (and men) are retraumatized in their experience of psychiatric care (Morrow, 2002).

Around the same time, a new administrator was hired at RVH who was willing to spearhead a process of institutional change that would involve staff training. Although this administrator had a feminist analysis of violence against women, she judged that the psychiatrists and other mental health professionals would not be comfortable actually addressing violence and sexual abuse in the lives of their patients. Nevertheless, the administrator invited me and another colleague[6] to participate in a process she hoped would result in training the staff at RVH becoming "trauma informed"—that is, the training would help staff recognize the impact of trauma on patients. Also, because the practices of psychiatry and institutionalization can themselves be traumatizing, we sought to prepare staff to recognize how routine practices (such as the use of constraints, and their own control over the daily activities of patients) could be changed to avoid harming those in care.

This process involved months of meetings with key staff members, including psychologists and nurses who headed particular units within the hospital. Only one psychiatrist actively participated in the process (she later told us that her own personal experience of working with clients who had revealed their sexual abuse histories was her motivation for participation). No other psychiatrists gave their support to the endeavor, although I was given space to present my research and the training initiative at "Doctor's Rounds," a monthly seminar for psychiatrists used to educate them about emerging research. The training process thus began on several wards, and a preliminary evaluation showed promising results in terms of shifting staff attitudes and practices.[7] Having no other real templates for how to carry out feminist change in psychiatric institutions, we did our best to bridge the divide between feminist analyses of violence and the ways that violence in women's lives has historically been either ignored or pathologized by psychiatry.

FEMINIST ANALYSIS AND ADVOCACY IN THE MENTAL HEALTH FIELD

The feminist critique of psychiatry first emerged during the resurgence of the women's movement in North America in the 1960s and 1970s. It began with women sharing their stories of abuse at the hands of psychiatry, and with the pivotal publication of American Phyllis Chesler's book *Women and Madness* (1972). Canadian feminist scholars also launched their own critique of the psychiatric paradigm (see, e.g., Penfold & Walker, 1983; Smith & David, 1975). These works comprehensively analyzed how madness has historically been rooted in normative ideas about femininity, and they exposed both the masculinist origins of psychiatry and the ways psychiatric treatment was structured to maintain and enforce women's subordination. Galvanized by this critique, activists and academics in the women's, psychiatric-survivor, and antipsychiatry movements became more vocal in their examination of women's experiences (Blackbridge & Gilhooly, 1985; Burstow & Weitz, 1988; Caplan, 1987; Kimball, 1975; Penfold & Walker, 1983; Woolsey, 1977). Only later, as the women's movement gained more currency and institutional power, did some feminists also begin to try to influence psychiatry and the mental health field from within, as I will show later.

Feminism, however, has had an "uneasy" relationship with psychiatric-survivor movements. Critics claim that the contemporary feminist movement is ignoring the voices and experiences of "psychiatrized"[8] women, and has sold out by adopting the discourses and practices of psychiatry and psychology (Burstow, 2005; Lamb, 1999). I will now try to grapple with the tensions arising from this critique and from the differing feminist positions on psychiatry, through a discussion of feminist attempts to have violence recognized as a precursor to mental health problems.

VIOLENCE AND MENTAL HEALTH

The prevalence and impact of violence against women has been a galva-nizing issue for the women's movement in North America and interna-tionally (Dobash & Dobash, 1992; Hankvisky & Varcoe, 2007; MacLeod, 1980). Indeed, the social and economic impacts of violence, as well as the many health and mental health consequences for individual women, have been widely documented (Campbell, 2002; Campbell, Woods, Chouaf, & Parker, 2000; UNIFEM, 2003; World Health Organization, 2002, 2004). For example, survivors of violence undergo more physi-cian and pharmacy visits, hospital stays, and mental health consulta-tions than other women do (Heise, Ellsberg, & Gottemoeller, 1999), and studies demonstrate that past and current experiences of intimate vio-lence are higher in both mental health inpatient and outpatient popu-lations than in the general female population (Beck & van der Kolk, 1987; Firsten, 1991; Fisher, 1998; Muenzenmaier, Mayer, & Struening, 1993). Researchers have also documented higher rates of substance use problems among women with co-occurring mental health problems and experiences of violence.[9]

At the same time, there have always been competing ideas within feminism about how best to understand male violence and, therefore, what kinds of solutions and strategies are most useful to stop it (Bonny-castle & Rigakos, 1998; MacLeod & DeKeseredy, 1997). For example, some recent feminist critics have argued that the hegemony of certain forms of feminism (liberal reformism) has resulted in the feminist anti-violence movement favoring institutional reforms and professionalized responses over more socially transformative strategies to end violence (Currie, 1998; Morrow, 1999; Walker, 1990). This debate is mirrored in feminist attempts to influence psychiatry and the mental health field.

RESPONSES TO VIOLENCE

Beginning with critical examinations of Freud's work on hysteria and his seduction theory, feminists and other scholars have documented how women's experiences of childhood sexual abuse, as well as their experiences of physical and sexual abuse as adults, historically have been disbelieved, downplayed, or used as evidence that they are "mad" (Astbury, 1996; Masson, 1986; Rush, 1980; Russell, 1986). In the early days of Canada's antiviolence movement (the 1970s and 1980s) feminists utterly rejected such psychiatrization of women who had experienced violence. When women who had been labeled mentally ill sought help from women's shelters and rape-crisis centers they were often encouraged to take part in activities of the women's movement and to see their own experiences in a social and political context. Thus, violence against women was understood by feminists as a political and social issue whose cure was radical social change involving challenges to patriarchal power within the family, and the dismantling of patriarchal and racist state institutions (Delacoste & Newman, 1981; Gupta & Makeda, 1983; MacLeod, 1980; Millet, 1970). Women's mental distress arising from violence was not something to be pathologized; it was seen as a normal and rational response to oppressive circumstances.

As the Canadian state apparatus began to pay more attention to violence against women and to fund shelters and rape-crisis centers in the mid 1980s, the function and mandate of these organizations evolved to conform to professional and bureaucratic practices, blunting feminist critiques and pulling the responses of feminists to women with mental health and substance-use problems more in line with the mainstream caring professions of social work, nursing, psychiatry, and psychology (Morrow, 1999; Morrow, Hankivsky, & Varcoe, 2004). The retrenchment of funding to women's organizations in the 1990s and 2000s (Bashevkin, 1998; Burt & Hardman, 2002; Burt & Mitchell, 1998) has further impacted the mandates and practices of women's organizations. For example, as women's organizations have come under increasing financial pressure, they have begun to screen women seeking protection and support more rigorously, with the aim of working only with those who strictly fit their mandate. This screening has included the use of psychiatric diagnostic labels to turn away women with mental illness or substance-use problems, now seen as best served elsewhere (or at least, as potentially depleting of limited resources).

At the same time, feminists have struggled to articulate the range of health/mental health effects of violence on women without buying into psychiatry wholesale. One strategy has been to frame violence as a health issue and thus engage health care professionals in the response to women who have experienced violence (Morrow & Varcoe, 2000). This is just one feminist tactic among several attempts to circumvent the power of psychiatry and other individualistic framings of violence, and arguably, it has helped to reshape health care responses to women.[10] Nonetheless, debate rages on. Hospital-based women-abuse programs have been lauded by some for helping to identify women who have been abused, but harshly criticized by others who argue that the screening tools used to identify abused women reinforce traditional health care models focused on the discernment of "cases," without providing the follow-up supports that might actually assist women in leaving violent relationships and/or addressing the underlying causes of violence (Dechief, 2003).

Feminists working within the psychiatric and psychological establishment have taken a similar tack—that of attempting to get women's experiences of sexual and physical abuse and the ensuing distress acknowledged within psychiatry. For example, they have pointed to the fact that there is a high level of correlation between certain psychiatric diagnoses (in particular, post-traumatic stress disorder and borderline-personality disorder) and experiences of childhood trauma and sexual abuse. They have made this connection in order to force a rethink of the cause of some women's mental health symptoms, and I would like to take time here to review their argument more carefully, in order to demonstrate further the challenges inherent in feminist efforts to change institutional practices in psychiatry from the inside.

The diagnostic label of post-traumatic stress disorder (PTSD) was first introduced into the *Diagnostic and Statistical Manual* (*DSM–IV–TR*)[11] in 1980 as a result of pressure from Vietnam veterans and their advocates, who were attempting to force recognition of the psychological effects of war-time trauma on men. Since this time the diagnostic criteria of PTSD have undergone several revisions, in part due to pressure from feminists who wanted the diagnosis to recognize traumas occurring more routinely in women's lives, primarily from physical and sexual abuse. The original articulation of PTSD indicated that the stressful events needed to be "outside the range of human experience," (Linder, 2000, p. 28) but feminists and others contested this and the criteria changed in the *DSM–IV–TR*, released in 2000 to include "normal" responses to stressful events. This opened the door for PTSD to be used as a diagnosis for women suffering the aftereffects of traumatic experiences including physical and sexual assault. Indeed, many feminist therapists consider the PTSD label one of the least problematic because it is one of the few diagnoses "whose symptoms can be said to stem from situational causes alone" (Becker, 2000, p. 422).

Nonetheless, critics have emerged to challenge the application of this diagnosis to abuse survivors. Some argue for an expansion of the criteria falling under the diagnosis of PTSD to capture a unique set of symptoms that result from early and chronic sexual abuse, such as feelings of powerlessness, disassociative symptoms, and self-blame (Herman, 1992; Wasserman & Rosenfeld, 1992). Herman (1992), for example, has lobbied to distinguish between different forms of trauma, suggesting a diagnostic category of "complex PTSD" for survivors of physical and sexual violence (p. 119). Therefore, the strategy of some feminists has been to work within psychiatry to expand and tweak diagnostic categories in order that they better capture women's experiences.

Others continue to challenge psychiatric diagnostic labeling wholesale (Becker, 2000; Lamb, 1999; Linder, 2004). For example, in her research, Linder (2004) found that clinicians' understandings of PTSD vary dramatically, and that empirical evidence has not been consistently used in backing diagnostic categories. Rather than seeing PTSD as too narrow a diagnosis, Linder (2004) argued that in effect PTSD has become "the catchall category for victims of trauma, including victims of domestic violence, sexual assault, and natural disasters" (p. 25).

In a similar vein, Becker (2000) contrasted PTSD with the diagnostic label of borderline-personality disorder (BPD), a label more frequently applied to women than to men. She characterizes BPD as the "bad girl" of psychiatric labels, in contrast to the "good girl"—PTSD (p. 422). While the label of PTSD is seen by some feminists as a breakthrough because it is a nonblaming diagnosis that acknowledges the social/structural origins of some mental health problems, BPD evokes the earlier diagnosis of hysteria, both because it is so frequently applied to women,[12] and because its "symptoms" are so varied and obscure (Becker, 2000). Although the role of trauma and violence in the etiology of BPD is increasingly recognized, the diagnosis of BPD is particularly stigmatizing. Among mental health professionals, women diagnosed with BPD are seen as some of the most difficult clients to work with, in part, because they are often "resistant" to treatment. As one psychiatrized women put it to me, "A diagnosis of BPD is like the kiss of death," (Anonymous, personal communication, 1999) since you are very likely going to be unable to access services (Morrow & Chappell, 1999). Indeed, access to public mental health care in Canada is based on screening practices that prioritize high acuity cases,[13] and often prevent people diagnosed with personality disorders from accessing care.

Becker (2000), in her comparative analysis of the diagnoses of BPD and PTSD, argued that the "stress paradigm" of illness reflected in PTSD serves to further medicalize women's responses to violence:

> As soon as we name a set of responses to stress 'disorder', we employ science to justify its medicalization. Not only, then, does acceptance of a reductionistic theoretical framework subordinate context to individual reaction, but medicalization further separates that reaction into its psychological and biological components. (p. 425)

It is useful to note here, however, that as prescient as the debates over labeling are—as well as being demonstrative of the conflicts between feminist critiques, with some seeking to transform the biomedical frame and some more radically rejecting it outright—they often exclude the actual voices of women who have carried these psychiatric labels. These women, more apt to belong to grassroots survivor movements, might well provide a more textured knowledge of how psychiatric discourses shape the lives of women and their self-understanding.

SOME CONCLUDING WORDS ON PSYCHIATRIC INSTITUTIONALIZATION AND "TRAUMA-INFORMED" CARE

The last part of the story of my experience of trying to influence the mental health practices at RVH (for the purposes of this chapter) is very much a reflection of the wider struggles and conflicts that have marked the history of women's mental health analysis, advocacy, and policy work, where a feminist structural analysis must often be strategically attenuated in order to make small inroads into medical and psychiatric practice. In the RVH example, in order to maintain our foothold in the institution, we labeled our work "trauma-informed" and purposely did not highlight the gendered nature of violence and sexual abuse in our approach to developing staff training.

Shortly after the introduction of our RVH staff training program in 2000, the province of British Columbia experienced a change of government that abruptly disrupted the project. The supportive administrator was fired, the supportive bureaucrat moved on to different responsibilities, and labor concerns began to take precedence as the government unrolled extensive new plans to downsize RVH. Unfortunately, the groundwork that was already set and the training that was already begun were lost as the policy direction shifted towards moving RVH patients to new locales throughout the province. In my view, this example illustrates both the possibilities for influencing change at the institutional level, and how vulnerable change processes are to the political process.

The changing policy context is, however, yielding new opportunities for interventions. For example, I am currently in the process of a 3-year study examining the final transfers of RVH's remaining occupants to towns throughout British Columbia and the ways gender and power relations play out in psychiatric institutions (see Morrow, Smith, Pederson, & Battersby, 2006).[14] These geographical transfers also involve a shift in the philosophy of care for people with mental illness—from a custodial model[15] to a psychosocial rehabilitation (PSR) model[16] that emphasizes recovery and personal autonomy. At the outset of this study I was hopeful that this shift might provide an opportunity to reintroduce the idea of trauma-informed care. However, preliminary analysis suggests that the PSR model is proving every bit as intransigent as traditional psychiatric care, since its focus on the individual does not allow a space for gendered or social analyses of people's experiences. As an example, in our interviews with psychiatrists and mental-health care providers, we are finding that attempts on the part of the interviewer to introduce a social analysis or to probe for gendered experiences are met with confusion, silence, or an assertion that people are treated as individuals, not as products of their social location.

Other kinds of initiatives outside psychiatric institutions are bringing different kinds of feminists together to work on providing better care to women-survivors of violence. For example, at the same time as the original RVH project was unfolding, the British Columbia Association of Specialized Victim Assistance and Counselling Programs (BCASVACP),[17] with involvement from British Columbia Yukon Transition House Society, or Transition House (an organization representing shelters across the province), began a cross-training initiative (entitled *Connecting: Mental Health and Violence Against Women*) in 1999, in response to concerns among their membership about working with women diagnosed with mental illness. This symposium was meant to facilitate knowledge exchange between mental health professionals and women working in antiviolence organizations. During the symposium, members of BCASVACP and Transition House workers came together with a group of feminist psychologists to share knowledge and discuss the challenges and possibilities of developing better programs for women.

It quickly became apparent, however, that the women in antiviolence organizations were working from very different assumptions than the feminist psychologists were. Antiviolence workers resisted the psychiatric labeling of women, and in feedback from participants after the fact, they complained that the knowledge exchange had only traveled one way: *from* feminist psychologists *to* antiviolence workers. The symposium thus highlighted how feminists working within different contexts and with different kinds of knowledge and training have dramatically differing understandings of women's lives and the relative merits of traditional psychiatric treatment.

Whether or not it may be deemed successful in the conventional sense of the term, the symposium represented, in microcosm, some of the divisions within feminism regarding how best to understand and work with women with mental health problems. I would argue that rather than weakening feminist claims, these divisions can help create a deeper appreciation for the complexity of the interactions between violence and mental distress, and that these examples of exchanges across feminist and mental health domains can teach us about how best to influence problematic psychiatric practices.

The increasingly frequent exchanges between mental health professionals and those located in antiviolence organizations, which result both from the general growth of feminist areas of critique, and the recent political and historical changes in the Canadian context as outlined in this chapter, are, in fact, leading to an emerging new language around trauma-informed and trauma-specific services, and to the development of programs that address the overlapping needs of women with violence, mental health, and substance-use issues. These programs are built on Canadian knowledge and programming (Haskell, 2001, 2003), including policy documents that argue for the benefits of integrative care (BC Ministry of Health Services, 2004; BCCEWH, 2004; Health Canada, 2001; Morrow 2003). Knowledge has also been gained from programs developed in the United States, for example, the seeking safety model developed by Lisa Najavits (Najavits, 1999), and the trauma, recovery, and empowerment model (TREM) developed by Maxine Harris (Harris, 1998). These models are currently being used and favorably evaluated in the *Women, Co-occurring Disorders and Violence Study* in the United States, launched in 1998, and sponsored by the Substance Abuse and Mental Health Services Administration (SAMHSA). The SAMHSA study is allowing communities to develop integrated approaches across a range of services, guided by a framework that is "gender specific, culturally competent, trauma-informed and trauma specific, comprehensive and integrated, and involve consumers/survivors/recovering persons (CSRs) in substantive and meaningful ways" (Veysey & Clark, 2004, p. 1).

On the one hand then, the development of practices and programs that address mental health and violence as interconnected lived experiences for women can be seen as progressive feminist interventions addressing the historical fragmentation of mental health and violence services, the continued dominance of biopsychiatry, and the lack of analysis regarding the impact of intimate violence on women's lives and of policy direction on these issues. It also speaks to the call from Ussher (1991) to move beyond feminist critiques of madness to constructive projects that acknowledge women's individual experiences of distress without compromising our understanding of the social and political contexts and the origins of these experiences of distress. The concern, however, is to maintain feminist structural analyses of violence in the context of a neoliberal climate that is drawn to individualistic framings of social and political concerns, and has resulted in a serious undermining of women's organizations and the social-welfare system. Certainly, the "psycho-pharmaceutical-industrial complex" is showing no signs of being tempered by structural understandings of human suffering, and arguably "trauma" is becoming a new buzzword, employed by the very institutional powers that have suppressed the acknowledgment of a connection between women's experiences of violence and their distress, something which signifies the need for "better" diagnoses, pharmaceutical solutions, and neuropsychological research, rather than the radical systemic change envisioned by feminists of the 1960s and 1970s (Levine, 2007). From this perspective, the continuing and changing role of feminist interventions is both essential, and fraught with challenges.

Several key questions continue to loom large: How is knowledge about women, mental illness, substance use, and violence produced? What are the social and institutional processes that shape the understanding of these issues, as information about them is exchanged? Specifically, what gets lost in translation when feminist activists and researchers (who couch these issues in social and political language) participate in knowledge-exchange processes that are meant to raise awareness of the issues and to engender health-system responses (and responses among other systems)? And, how do the competing needs and relative power of information-exchange players affect those responses?

RECONSTRUCTING MADNESS

As Benedict Carey asked in 2005, writing in the *New York Times* about the recent release of a government-sponsored survey on mental health (the most comprehensive U.S. survey to date, and one that predicts that more than half of all Americans will develop a mental disorder in their lives):

> But what does it mean when more than half of a society may suffer 'mental illness'? Is it an indictment of modern life or a sign of greater willingness to deal openly with a once-taboo subject? Or is it another example of the American mania to give every problem a name, a set of symptoms and a treatment—a trend, medical historians say, accentuated by drug marketing to doctors and patients?

The Canadian landscape is no different: the main strategy of mental-health-advocacy organizations has been to reduce the stigma of mental illness by likening it to physical-health ailments, effectively erasing any of the social context in which mental distress occurs, and blunting any critique of diagnostic practices.[18] In this context, feminist interventions notwithstanding, diagnoses like PTSD and BPD are widely applied to all sorts of symptoms and experiences, and structural analyses of these traumas remain largely submerged. In such an environment, labeling women "vulnerable" and "victimized" is acceptable, while resistance strategies that challenge gender, race, and class hierarchies are not.

Feminists have not always been immune to this "syndromizing" of experience, and, as these new directions in policy and practice unfold, we must remain vigilant towards "progressive" innovations that may themselves come to replicate the very medicalization/categorization they were designed to undermine. Becker (2000) said,

Paradoxically, trauma focused therapy fits well into the medical model, notwithstanding its proponents' views and sentiments to the contrary. When trauma is centralized, not only do medical metaphors such as wound, injury, brokenness and pain pervade the language of the therapeutic encounter, but healing and recovery become the goals of psychotherapy. (p. 430)

As more initiatives bring feminists and mental-health care professionals together, independence of language and approach will be central. Feminists must remain wary of the temptation to adopt the language of power (psychiatry) in order to gain recognition. Any reconstructive project must balance women's individual experiences of distress with the social against the political origins of this distress. One way of maintaining vigilance is to constantly engage the "subjugated" and "local" knowledges of psychiatrized women in devising strategies for interventions into psychiatry, and to form alliances with psychiatric-survivor movements that are attempting to have the rights of people with mental illness recognized and respected. While the institution of psychiatry appears to remain impervious to activist demands, especially on the question of violence against women, small gains are being made by feminists who are extending their analysis of violence as a health issue into developing interventions based in women's organizations and involving feminist mental health workers.

REFERENCES

American Psychiatric Association. (2000). *Diagnostic and statistical manual of mental disorders text revisions* (4th ed.). American Psychiatric Association.

Astbury, J. (1996). *Crazy for you: The making of women's madness.* New York: Oxford University Press.

Bashevkin, S. (1998). *Women on the defensive.* Chicago: University of Chicago Press.

BC Ministry of Health Services (2004). *Every door is the right door: A BC planning framework to address problem substance use and addiction.* Victoria, Canada: Ministry of Health Services.

BCCEWH. (2004). *Advancing the health of girls and women: A provincial women's health strategy.* Vancouver, Canada: BC Women's Hospital and the BC Centre of Excellence for Women's Health.

Beck, J., & van der Kolk, B. (1987). Reports of childhood incest and current behavior of chronically hospitalized psychotic women. *American Journal of Psychiatry, 144,* 1474–1476.

Becker, D. (2000). When she was bad: Borderline personality disorder in a posttraumatic age. *American Journal of Orthopsychiatry, 70*(4), 422–432.

Blackbridge, P., & Gilhooly, S. (1985). *Still sane.* Vancouver, Canada: Press Gang.

Bonnycastle, K., & Rigakos, G. (Eds.). (1998). *Unsettling truths: Battered women, policy, politics and contemporary research in Canada.* Vancouver, Canada: Collective Press.

Burstow, B. (2005). Feminist antipsychiatry praxis—Women and the movement(s): A Canadian perspective. In W. Chan, D. Chunn, & R. Menzies (Eds.), *Women, madness and the law: A feminist reader* (pp. 245–258). London: Glasshouse.

Burstow, B., & Weitz, D. (Eds.) (1988). *Shrink resistant: The struggle against psychiatry in Canada.* Vancouver, Canada: New Star.

Burt, S., & Hardman, S. (2002). The case of disappearing targets: The Liberals and gender equality. In L. Pal (Ed.), *How Ottawa spends 2001–2002: Power in transition* (pp. 201–222). Toronto: Oxford University Press.

Burt, S., & Mitchell, C. (1998). What's in a name? From sheltering women to protecting communities. In L. Pal (Ed.), *How Ottawa spends 2001–2002: Power in transition* (pp. 271–291). Toronto: Oxford University Press.

Campbell, J. (2002). Health consequences of intimate partner violence. *The Lancet, 359,* 1331–1336.

Campbell, J., Woods, A., Chouaf, K., & Parker, B. (2000). Reproductive health consequences of intimate partner violence: A nursing research review. *Clinical Nursing Research, 9*(3), 217–237.

Caplan, P. (1987). *The myth of women's masochism.* Scarborough, Canada: New American Library of Canada.

Caplan, P., & Cosgrove, L. (Eds.). (2004). *Bias in psychiatric diagnoses.* New York: The Rowman and Littlefield Publishing Group.

Carey, B. (2005, July 12). Who is mentally ill? Deciding is often all in the mind. *New York Times.* Retrieved June 2006, from http://www.nytimes.com/2005/06/12/weekinreview/12carey.html

Chesler, P. (1972). *Women and madness.* New York: Avon Books.

Corker, M., & Shakespeare, T. (2002). Mapping the terrain. In M. Corker & T. Shakespeare (Eds.), *Disability/postmodernity: Embodying disability theory* (pp. 1–17). London: Continuum.

Cosgrove, L., Krimsky, S., Vijayaraghavan, M., & Schneider, L. (2006). Financial ties between DSM–IV panel members and the pharmaceutical industry. *Psychotherapy and Psychosomatics, 73*(3), 154–160.

Craine, L., Henson, C., & Colliver, J. (1988). Prevalence of a history of sexual abuse among female psychiatric patients in a state hospital system. *Hospital and Community Psychiatry, 39,* 300–304.

Currie, D. (1998). The criminalization of violence against women: Feminist demands and patriarchal accommodation. In K. Bonnycastle & G. Rigakos (Eds.), *Unsettling truths: Battered women, policy, politics and contemporary research in Canada* (pp. 41–51). Vancouver, Canada: Collective Press.

Dechief, L. (2003). *Care, control and connection: Health care experiences of women in abusive intimate relationships.* Unpublished Master of Science thesis. University of British Columbia, Vancouver, Canada.

Delacoste, F., & Newman, F. (Eds.) (1981). *Fight back! Feminist resistance to male violence.* Minneapolis, MN: Cleis Press.

Devault, M., & McCoy, L. (2002). Institutional ethnography: Using interviews to investigate ruling relations. In F. Gubrium & J. Holstein (Eds.), *Handbook of interview research: Context and method* (pp. 751–775). Thousand Oaks, CA: Sage.

Diamond, I., & Quinby, L (Eds.) (1988). *Feminism and Foucault: Reflections on resistance.* Boston: North Eastern University Press.

Diedrich, L. (2007). Cultures of dis/ability: From being stigmatized to doing disability. In M. Morrow, O. Hankivsky, & C. Varcoe (Eds.), *Women's health in Canada: Critical perspectives on theory and policy* (pp. 244–271). Toronto, Canada: University of Toronto Press.

Dobash, R., & Dobash, R. (1992). *Women, violence and social change.* New York: Routledge.

Dreyfus, H., & Rabinow, P. (1982). *Michel Foucault: Beyond structuralism and hermeneutics.* Chicago: University of Chicago Press.

Firsten, T. (1991). Violence in the lives of women on psychiatric wards. *Canadian Woman's Studies/les cahiers de la femme, 11*(4), 45–48.

Fisher, P. (1998). Women and mental health issues: The role of trauma [Special issue on womens's mental health]. *Visions: BC's Mental Health Journal, 3,* 7.

Ford, M., & Widiger, T. (1989, April). Sex bias in the diagnosis of histrionic and antisocial personality disorders. *Journal of Consulting and Clinical Psychology, 57*(2), 301–305.

Foucault, M. (2003). *Society must be defended: Lectures at the College de France 1975–1976.* New York: Picador.

Gupta, N., & Makeda, S. (1983). *The issue is "ism": Women of colour speak out.* Toronto, Canada: Sister Vision.

Hankivsky, O., & Varcoe, C. (2007). From global to local and over the rainbow: Violence against women. In M. Morrow, O. Hankivsky, & C. Varcoe (Eds.), *Women's health in Canada: Critical perspectives on theory and policy* (pp. 477–506). Toronto, Canada: University of Toronto Press.

Harris, M. (1998). *Trauma, recovery and empowerment: A clinician's guide for working with women in groups.* New York: The Free Press.

Haskell, L. (2001). *Bridging responses: A front-line worker's guide to supporting women who have post-traumatic stress.* Toronto, Canada: Centre for Addiction and Mental Health.

Haskell, L. (2003). *First stage trauma treatment: A guide for therapists working with women.* Toronto, Canada: Centre for Addictions and Mental Health.

Health Canada. (2001). *Best practices: Concurrent mental health and substance use disorders.* Ottawa, Canada: Health Canada.

Heise, L., Ellsberg M., & Gottemoeller, M. (1999). *Ending violence against women.* (Population Information Program. Series L, No. 11.) Johns Hopkins University School of Public Health, Baltimore.

Herman, J. (1992). *Trauma and recovery.* New York: HarperCollins.

Kimball, M. (1975). Sex role stereotypes and mental health: Catch 22. In D. Smith & S. David (Eds.), *Women look at psychiatry* (pp. 121–142). Vancouver, Canada: Press Gang.

Kirby, M. (2006, May). *Out of the shadows at last: Transforming mental health, mental illness and addiction services in Canada 2006. Final report of the Standing Senate Committee on Social Affairs, Science and Technology.* Ottawa, Canada: The Standing Senate Committee on Social Affairs, Science and Technology.

Lamb, S. (1999). Constructing the victim popular images and lasting labels. In S. Lamb (Ed.), *New versions of victims: Feminists struggle with the concept* (pp. 108–138). New York: New York University Press.

Levine, B. (2007, November 1). The U.S. psycho-pharmaceutical industrial complex: As mental illness has become profitable, we are seeing more of it. *Z Magazine*. Retrieved March 3, 2008, from http://www.zcommunications.org/zmag/viewArticle/15950

Linder, M. (2004). Creating post-traumatic stress disorder: A case study of the history, sociology, and politics of psychiatric classification. In P. Caplan & L. Cosgrove (Eds.), *Bias in psychiatric diagnosis* (pp. 25–40). New York: The Rowman and Littlefield Publishing Group.

MacLeod, L. (1980). *Wife battering in Canada: The vicious circle*. Ottawa, Canada: Advisory Council on the Status of Women.

MacLeod, L., & DeKeseredy, W. (1997). *Woman abuse: A sociological story*. Toronto, Canada: Harcourt Brace and Co.

Masson, J. (1986). *A dark science: Women, sexuality and psychiatry in the nineteenth century*. New York: Farrar, Straus, and Giroux.

Millet, K. (1970). *Sexual politics*. Garden City, NY: Double Day and Co.

Morrow, M. (1999). Feminist anti-violence activism: Organizing for change. In S. Brodribb (Ed.), *Reclaiming the future: Women's strategies for the 21st century* (pp. 237–257). Charlottetown, Canada: Gynergy Books.

Morrow, M. (2002). *Violence and trauma in the lives of women with serious mental illness: Current practices in service provision in British Columbia*. Vancouver, Canada: British Columbia Centre of Excellence for Women's Health.

Morrow, M. (2003). *Mainstreaming women's mental health: Building a Canadian strategy*. Vancouver, Canada: British Columbia Centre of Excellence for Women's Health.

Morrow, M., & Chappell, M. (1999). *Hearing women's voices: Mental health care for women*. Vancouver, Canada: British Columbia Centre of Excellence for Women's Health.

Morrow, M., Hankivsky, O., & Varcoe, C. (2004). Women and violence: The effects of dismantling the welfare state. *Journal of Critical Social Policy, 24*(3), 358–384.

Morrow, M., & Varcoe, C. (2000). *Violence against women: Improving the health care response—A guide for health authorities, health care managers, providers and planners.* Victoria, Canada: Ministry of Health.

Morrow, M., Smith, J., Pederson, A., & Battersby, L. (2006, spring) Relocations, dislocations and innovations in mental health reform: Examining the impact of psychiatric deinstitutionalization on women, men and communities. *Research Bulletin,* 5(1), 19–20. Retrieved from http://www.cewh-cesf.ca/en/publications/RB/v5n1/page9.shtml

Muenzenmaier, K., Mayer E., & Struening, E. (1993). Childhood abuse and neglect among women outpatients with chronic mental illness. *Hospital and Community Psychiatry, 44,* 666–670.

Najavits, L. (1999). Seeking safety: A new cognitive-behavioral therapy for PTSD and substance abuse. *National Center for Post-Traumatic Stress Disorder Clinical Quarterly, 8*(3), 40–45.

Penfold, P., & Walker, G. (1983). *Women and the psychiatric paradox.* Montreal, Canada: Eden Press.

Rush, F. (1980). *The best kept secret: Sexual abuse of children.* Upper Saddle River, NJ: Prentice-Hall.

Russell, D. (1986). *The secret trauma: Incest in the lives of girls and women.* New York: Basic Books.

Sawicki, J. (1998). Feminism, Foucault and "subjects" of power and freedom. In J. Moss (Ed.), *The later Foucault: politics and philosophy* (pp. 93–107). Thousand Oaks, CA: Sage Publications.

Smith, D. (2005). *Institutional ethnography: A sociology for people.* Victoria, Canada: University of Victoria Press.

Smith, D., & David, S. (Eds.). (1975). *Women look at psychiatry.* Vancouver, Canada: Press Gang.

UNIFEM. (2003). *Not a minute more.* New York: United Nations Development Fund for Women.

Ussher, J. (1991). *Women's madness: Misogyny or mental illness?* Amherst, MA: The University of Massachusetts Press.

Veysey, B., & Clark, C. (2004). Responding to physical and sexual abuse in women with alcohol and other drug and mental disorders: Program building. *Alcoholism Treatment Quarterly, 22*(3/4), 1–18.

Walker, G. (1990). *Family violence and the women's movement: The conceptual politics of struggle.* Toronto, Canada: University of Toronto Press.

Wasserman, S., & Rosenfeld, A. (1992). An overview of the history of child sexual abuse and Sigmund Freud's contributions. In W. O'Donohue & J. Geer (Eds.), *The sexual abuse of children: Theory and research* (pp. 49–72). Hillsdale, NJ: Lawrence Erlbaum Associates.

Widiger, T., & Weissman, M. (1991) Epidemiology of borderline personality disorder. *Hospital and Community Psychiatry, 42,* 1015–1021.

Woolsey, L. (1977). Psychology and the reconciliation of women's double bind: To be feminine or to be fully human. *Canadian Psychological Review, 18*(1), 66–78.

World Health Organization (WHO). (2002). *World report on violence and health: Update.* Geneva, Switzerland: Author.

World Health Organization (WHO). (2004). *The economic dimensions of interpersonal violence.* Geneva, Switzerland: Author, Department of Injuries and Violence Prevention.

1. The antipsychiatry movement has its roots in critiques of psychiatry launched in the 1960s and 1970s, mainly by academics, some of whom were themselves trained as psychiatrists. Psychiatric-survivor movements are those that originate in the psychiatric system, and are led by people who have been there. These people variously refer to themselves as "consumers," "consumer-survivors," "ex-patients," and "psychiatric survivors." These individuals have varying positions on psychiatry, but have all fought for the recognition of their right to be involved in their own treatment and to decrease discrimination and stigma against people with mental illness. For a recent discussion of these movements, see Burstow (2005).

2. Here and throughout this chapter I use the term "mental illness" with an awareness of its contested nature. That is, scholars and activists concerned with the construction of madness often reject the label of "illness," in part because it serves to medicalize or pathologize experiences that could otherwise be seen as "normal" or "understandable" reactions to life events and stresses. In view of this I sometimes substitute "mental distress" for "mental illness."

3. Although violence against women has been used to describe a wide array of actions against women, including political and social violence, in this context I am referring primarily to the intimate forms of violence women experience, usually at the hands of the men they know, that is, sexual abuse as a child, and violence in the context of an intimate relationship.

4. Trauma-informed services are those that provide care with an awareness of the potential effects of violence and therefore try to be sensitive to and minimize those effects. Trauma-specific services directly address the effects of violence on individuals, usually through individual therapy and/or peer support groups.

5. RVH was, until recently, the only provincial tertiary-care psychiatric facility in British Columbia. Historically, it admitted "patients" diagnosed as mentally ill from all over British Columbia into its care. At one time RVH housed approximately 5,000 people. It has since gone through successive rounds of downsizing and, in the current regionalized health care system, which aims to decentralize care in this geographically immense province, the remaining occupants (about 400–500 people) are being transferred to facilities in other cities and towns throughout British Columbia.

6. I want to acknowledge the work of Kathleen Whipp, the counselor/educator/ trainer who developed trauma-informed programming for RVH, based on the work of Maxine Harris (1998).

7. The evaluation was conducted by Nancy Poole at the British Columbia Centre of Excellence for Women's Health, but was never published.

8. The term "psychiatrization" is used to describe people's negative experiences with psychiatry.

9. It should be noted that there is a large body of feminist literature on the intersections of substance use and violence, some of which also addresses mental health issues. Examples include the following: "Women's Pain: Working With Women Concurrently on Substance Use, Experience of Trauma and Mental Health Issues [Special issue: Concurrent Disorders, Mental Disorders and Substance Abuse]," by N. Poole, 2004, *Visions: BC's Mental Health and Addictions Journal, 2*, pp. 29–32; "The Link Between Substance Abuse and Post-traumatic stress disorder in women: A research review, by L. M. Najavits, R. D. Weiss, and S. R. Shaw, 1997, *American Journal of Addiction, 6*, pp. 273–283; and "Creating Trauma Services for Women with Co-Occurring Disorders: Experiences from the SAMHSA Women With Alcohol, Drug Abuse and Mental Health Disorders Who Have Histories of Violence Study," by D. J. Moses, B. Glover-Reed, R. Mazelis, and B. D' Ambrosio, August 2003, retrieved April 6, 2008, from http://www.prainc.com/wcdvs/publications/default.asp

10. The Woman Abuse Program at British Columbia Women's Hospital, which trains health professionals to identify and respond to women who have experiences of violence, is a good example of transformed institutional responses resulting from this framing.

11. Psychiatric diagnosis is accomplished through the use of the *DSM*, a classification system of mental "disorders" developed by the American Psychiatric Association (APA). The *DSM* has undergone four revisions since its inception in 1968, with the next due in 2011. At every step, controversy has surrounded its development and use. Critics charge that the method used to develop the criteria for the *DSM* is unscientific, that deeply held sexist and racist biases influence diagnostic criteria (see Caplan & Cosgrove, 2004; Ford & Widiger, 1989), and that links between the experts who determine diagnostic criteria and the pharmaceutical industry are too close for the development of objective criteria (Cosgrove, Krimsky, Vijayaraghavan, & Schneider, 2006).

12. BPD is applied to women at a rate of 7 women to 1 man (Widiger & Weissman, 1991).

13. Acuity is determined by a number of factors, including psychiatric diagnosis and the degree of functional impairment experienced by the individual. In a system with scarce resources, however, diagnosis is sometimes used to screen out individuals for care. For example, most mental health teams in British Columbia take clients with axis I diagnoses, such as schizophrenia and major affective disorders, and may not routinely take clients with axis II diagnoses, such as personality disorders. For a description of axes I and II see American Psychiatric Association (2000).

14. This study employs Dorothy Smith's institutional ethnography (Smith, 2005). Smith, like Foucault, is interested in "texts, power and governance," but the method of institutional ethnography focuses more on the actual activities of individuals and how they activate "texts" (Devault and McCoy, 2002, p. 772).

15. Custodial care is typified by the idea that people with mental illness can only be stabilized, and ultimately, will never recover. They must thus be cared for in long-stay institutions where their lives are continuously regulated by care aids and mental health professionals.

16. The use of psychosocial rehabilitation models in mental health is not new. However, these have been especially difficult to implement in large psychiatric institutions where traditions of custodial care dominate and where paternalistic institutional practices are often entrenched.

17. The BCASVACP is a provincial organization that has provided a communication network among community-based victim-assistance programs, sexual-assault centers, and Stopping the Violence counselling programs.

18. This is the tack taken by the recently released report from the Canadian Standing Senate Committee on Social Affairs, Science, and Technology by Senator Michael Kirby (see Kirby, 2006).

CHAPTER 7

GLOBALIZATION, TRAFFICKING, AND HEALTH:

A CASE STUDY OF UKRAINE

Olena Hankivsky

INTRODUCTION

As a country of origin and transit point, Ukraine has one of the worst human-trafficking problems in Europe. Many of those affected are women trafficked into the sex trade. The extent of the problem has drawn international attention, with various agencies and governments weighing in on the Ukrainian government's response to the issue. What has been missing from many of these evaluations to date, however, is the extent to which external forces bear upon current circumstances inside Ukraine. Evidently, destination countries create the demand for trafficking. In many cases, they enable conditions for it to flourish. Moreover, the international community has considerable influence over the creation and transmission of knowledge regarding sex trafficking, which, in turn, shapes how the issue is framed locally, and what policy responses are developed.

In Ukraine, this means most efforts are focused on describing the problem, identifying the players involved, revealing trafficking routes and practices, and offering legal solutions and recommendations for how to combat the problem (Hughes & Denisova, 2001), sometimes to the exclusion of other possible policy directions. Also, the increasingly dominant conceptualization of trafficking as primarily a human-rights issue on the international scene is crowding out alternative framings and concomitant policy responses at the national level. There is very little discussion of exactly how international forces contribute to the prioritization of certain perspectives and information that lead to a narrow conceptualization of a phenomenon that is actually complex, multifaceted, and multinational.

In this chapter I will challenge the assumption that internal failings of the Ukrainian government and state are fully responsible for that country's apparently incomplete understanding of trafficking, and the inadequate policy responses to trafficking across sectors. Rather, I will suggest that Ukraine's response is a manifestation of links between economic globalization, market reforms, and the emergence and growth of human trafficking, as well as the relationship between trafficking, gender, and women's health. A result of this is that the health needs of trafficked women have been pushed down the agenda, despite the fact that physical- and mental health consequences are not simply side effects of trafficking, but issues central to it. In conclusion, I will propose that unless information on the scope of trafficking is brought to the fore, and the international community shifts its priorities and values in relation to economic globalization in order to move beyond the hegemony of human-rights discourse, origin and transit countries like Ukraine will be greatly compromised in their ability to work across borders to develop effective prevention and intervention initiatives to deal with sex trafficking.

TRAFFICKING

Although there is no agreement on the definition of trafficking in human beings, many countries and reports draw on protocols of the United Nations Convention against Transnational Organized Crime, in which trafficking in persons is characterized as

> the recruitment, transportation, transfer, harbouring or receipt of persons, by means of the threat or use of force or other forms of coercion, of abduction, of fraud, of deception, of the abuse of power or of a position of vulnerability or of the giving or receiving of payments or benefits to achieve the consent of a person having control over another person, for the purposes of exploitation. Exploitation shall include, at a minimum, the exploitation of the prostitution of others or other forms of sexual exploitation, forced labour or services, slavery or practices similar to slavery, servitude or the removal of organs. (United Nations, 2000, p. 32)

It has only been in the past 5 years, however, that the worldwide problem of trafficking has found a priority position on the agendas of nation states and a range of international and state organizations. The United States, for example, sees itself as an international leader in this area. On the occasion of the release of the 5th annual U.S. Department of State "Trafficking in Persons Report," Condoleeza Rice stated,

> Trafficking in human beings is nothing less than a modern form of slavery. And President Bush has called upon all countries to confront this evil. As the President has said, "human life is the gift of our Creator and it should never be for sale." The United States has a particular duty to fight this scourge because trafficking in persons is an affront to the principles of human dignity and liberty, upon which this nation was founded. (U.S. Department of State, 2005, n.p.)

According to the International Organization for Migration (IOM), sex trafficking is estimated to be a $6–12 billion industry (Time International, 2001). Women and men are trafficked from within developing and transitional countries to both developing and developed countries and regions with sex industries, including Western Europe, the United States, Australia, and Canada. Approximately 700,000–1.5 million women and children are trafficked across international borders annually (IOM, 2001), and globalization, along with looser travel restrictions in some jurisdictions, has made it easier for traffickers to transport women and children across borders (UNICEF, 2001).

The theoretical frame for analyzing trafficking includes seeing this problem as a moral, criminal, migration, public-order, or human-rights issue (Bruckert & Parent, 2002). The links between economic globalization, gender, and health in the context of sex trafficking, however, remain largely uninvestigated in both research and policy. Even though the trafficking of women and girls is arguably one of the most significant trends associated with the current wave of globalization (Maclean & Sicchia, 2004), adequate research has not been undertaken to illuminate the core reasons for this problem, or how it relates specifically to gender and health. In Ukraine, there is both a lack of knowledge about trafficking in general and its gendered health dimensions. This is compounded by a general lack of awareness of trafficking's health consequences among all segments of the population.

UKRAINE AND TRAFFICKING

According to the IOM (1995), "until 1992 there were virtually no known cases of trafficked women from Central and Eastern Europe" (p. 6). Although reliable data is not always available, it is estimated that over 100,000 women are trafficked internationally each year from the former Soviet Union (Miko & Park, 2003). In the sex industry, because they are often tall, slim, and blond, women from Russia and Ukraine are considered to be the most valuable (Hughes, 2001). Traffickers in Ukraine receive between US$800 and $11,000 per woman delivered to pimps abroad, making it a lucrative business for those involved (Hughes, 2001). The most popular destination countries are Canada, China, the Czech Republic, France, Germany, Greece, Hungary, Israel, Italy, Korea, The Netherlands, Poland, Portugal, Russia, Spain,

Switzerland, Syria, Turkey, the United Arab Emirates, the United States, and Yugoslavia.

In general, the collapse of the Soviet Union created ideal conditions for the trafficking of women: open borders for travel, increased migration, and privatized trade. In Ukraine, these have been further distilled: increased economic globalization has resulted in the entrenchment and growth of shadow economies and criminal networks (Hughes, 2001). In 2000, the World Bank reported that the trafficking of women from Ukraine into forced labor "has reached an unprecedented level even when compared to other Former Soviet Union countries" (quoted in Rasner, 2004). Ukraine's Interior Ministry has reported that up to 400,000 women under the age of 30 have left in the last decade (IOM, 2001), a significant number of them through trafficking. It is estimated that every tenth Ukrainian has someone close who has fallen victim to human trafficking (RISU, 2005). Despite numerous educational antitrafficking campaigns, many women continue to look for ways to leave the country (Uehling, 2004).

Women from 18 to 25 years old are most at risk in terms of sex trafficking, as are women from rural areas (Rudd, 2002) and young girls leaving state orphanages (Lutsenko, Matiaszek, Scanlan, & Shab, 2005). These women are willing to "work abroad illegally; leave Ukraine without a visa, even if this means endangering their personal welfare; work in the sex industry; work abroad as dancers and striptease; trust agencies that provide matrimonial matches with foreigners" (Winrock International, 2001, p. 3). Among those actively recruited for work abroad, the majority receive propositions from relatives, friends, and acquaintances rather than recruitment firms or strangers. As Pyshchulina (2005) explained,

> It is difficult to reduce or eliminate the trafficking web, as it involves not only organized crime circles that have found a profitable source of income second only to drug and arms trafficking, but also a whole network of intermediaries who subtly work between family and friends. (p. 117)

In addition to this, recruitment often takes place through an organization, which, "functioning in a similar manner to a job placement agency that facilitates irregular migration, may not appear any different from legitimate services arranging successful migrations" (Lutsenko et al., 2005, p. 43). Sophisticated deception is thus a crucial strategy in trafficking (Hughes & Denisova, 2001; Uehling, 2004).

There are also important "push" factors related to the current socio-economic situation and the declining standard of living for Ukrainian women (Lakiza-Sachuk, 2003). The last report submitted by the Government of Ukraine on the status of the implementation of initiatives under the Convention on the Elimination of all forms of Discrimination Against Women (CEDAW) highlights the grave economic situation of Ukrainian women.

After the collapse of the Soviet Union, it was mostly women who lost their employment. More than two thirds of unemployed people in Ukraine are women (von Struensee, 2000). Discrimination in the labor market is systemic, even in the public sector (Lutsenko et al., 2005). Economically, the burden of transitioning to a market economy weighs more heavily on women than men, particularly because of the decline of social and public services, occurring alongside growing unemployment and higher inflation. In an atmosphere of deepening poverty and widening social inequalities, women face the triple burden of high unemployment, job discrimination, and a permissive attitude toward sexual harassment in the workplace. It is consistently reported that women who look for work abroad "seek to overcome poverty, to improve their financial status and live better than their parents did" (Winrock International, 2001, p. 5). Of course, the "myth of an easy and affluent life in the West...also contributes to the phenomenon" (Pyshchulina 2005, p. 116).

Most of the available information about the experience of being trafficked comes from women who return home, come forward, and seek assistance, rather than those who cannot return or choose not to. It is worth highlighting that the risks involved in migrating abroad for employment are quite widely recognized. One recent study reported that "78% [of women] knew of the dangers of working abroad, including the possibility of being cheated by employers and middlemen who offer passage to work abroad" (Winrock International, 2001, p. 6). This does not, however, correlate with equal awareness about trafficking, and how it is linked to a transition abroad in search of work. According to both women who want to go abroad to work and those who have returned, scant knowledge of either the legalities of foreign employment, or the possible consequences of illegal migration is a factor in the spread of the trafficking problem in Ukraine. For example, in the same study mentioned above, only 38% of the women reported knowing about the dangers of becoming a victim of trafficking in women, and less than half (48%) reported being aware of the risks of having their passport seized or having fictitious debt created by their employer in order to recruit and maintain them as sex slaves (Winrock International, p. 6).

Once entrapped in the sex industry, women have very few exit options as they endure violence, rape, threats to themselves and their families, and debt bondage. In her examination of women from Eastern Europe who are trafficked to Greece, Lazaridis (2001) explained that there are only four ways to escape from trafficking: becoming unprofitable to pimps because of emotional breakdown; becoming unprofitable to pimps because of advance stage of pregnancy; being helped to escape by a client; and death. Significantly, many do not have access to medical care. In some instances, when a woman becomes ill, she is simply killed by her captors (Miko & Park, 2003). Moreover, the countries where the women find themselves provide little support, often treating them as criminals and prostitutes. For those women who do find a way to return home, only 12% report their victimization (Hughes & Denisova, 2001). Very few girls and young women are aware of NGOs that assist women who have been victims of trafficking (Winrock International, 2001).

Internal Responses
At the grassroots level in Ukraine, numerous NGOs have worked hard to assist victims of trafficking, and have lobbied government for new legislation, programs, and other initiatives. One noteworthy example is La Strada: The International Women's Rights Center, established in 1997, which has been central in developing information and lobby campaigns, prevention-education campaigns, social-assistance campaigns,

and establishing a La Strada Hotline.[1] Presently, there are over 25 NGOs working on countertrafficking initiatives, and in the last few years, they have been responsible for over 1,800 victims of trafficking being reunited with their families (Kateryna Cherepakha, personal correspondence, September 2005).

In recent years, drawing on international conventions and human-rights discourse, the Ukrainian government has taken concrete steps to improve the status of women, reverse the emigration of women, and combat trafficking. The Ministry of Family, Children, and Youth Affairs and the Ministry of Internal Affairs play key roles in overseeing a range of antitrafficking initiatives, including the Comprehensive Program for Combating Trafficking. Appendix D consists of a chronology detailing some of the more important developments, and is helpful in illustrating the state's priorities (see appendices section at the back of this book).

Policy makers and international donors routinely divide trafficking interventions into three categories: prosecution, protection and assistance, and prevention. In Ukraine, in terms of the first of these, the criminal code remains inadequate to address the full range of trafficking practices, or to arrest and prosecute the greatest number of international traffickers, in part because the code definition does not cover trafficking within the country's borders. Few cases related to trafficking in humans are prosecuted to the full extent of the law. Trafficking-related complicity and official involvement continue to be a problem; high-level official intervention to prevent smooth legal proceedings against traffickers has been documented. Indeed, "widespread corruption…affects all levels of society, including policy, prosecutors, and judges" (Pyshchulina, 2005, p. 117).

The government also fails to provide adequate protection and rehabilitation services for victims of trafficking, who are often intimidated and threatened, and will thus refuse to testify. Those who do testify are consistently treated with a lack of sensitivity; many are characterized as prostitutes instead of victims of serious crimes. As Pyshchulina (2005) explained, the "absence of witness protection and procedural safeguards for victims or witnesses during criminal proceedings, especially with regard to the protection and privacy and safety of the victim" (p. 120) greatly impairs the government's ability to protect victims. These weaknesses are also reflected in Ukraine's prevention efforts. The government continues to rely on NGOs and international organizations, including UNICEF, IOM, USAID, the British Council, and OSCE, to fund and conduct the bulk of prevention programs, a factor contributing to the dominance of discourses adhered to by those organizations in Ukraine, as will be discussed later in this chapter.

Most importantly, the country's Comprehensive Program for Combating Trafficking (Comprehensive Program), which focuses on raising awareness of trafficking in human beings, improving economic opportunities and awareness of rights, supervising migration, and reducing risk factors, has had only a very limited impact. While no one program could bring about all the required changes, its efficacy has been undermined by the lack of much-needed socioeconomic changes. Compared to other former Soviet countries, Ukraine lags behind in economic and political reforms (Pyshchulina, 2005, p. 116). As Pyshchulina explained, "The prolonged political and socioeconomic transition has had severe implications, including the marginalization and, to some extent, exclusion of some groups from the social and political forefront. One of these groups is women" (p. 116). While the Orange Revolution and the election of President Yushchenko held great promise of democratic reform in Ukraine—indeed, early in his term, trafficking was made a priority issue—the rise in shadow economies and the strength of transnational criminal networks continue to compound the vulnerability of Ukrainian women. Moreover, as the U.S. Department of State (2007) recently concluded, corruption in Ukraine leads to the complicity in trafficking by government officials.

The shortcomings of current internal efforts have led to numerous recommendations regarding how Ukraine can improve its response to sex trafficking. For instance, a 2005 report coproduced by UNICEF, OSCE, USAID, and the British Council, entitled *Trafficking in Ukraine: An Assessment of Current Responses*, makes 40 recommendations that address a range of shortcomings across sectors and begins to raise the issue of the role the international community (and specifically destination countries) has in reducing trafficking and better supporting Ukraine. In the same year, the U.S. Department of State summarized its assessment of the Ukrainian efforts by concluding that

> the government should create a special witness protection program for trafficking victims, expand the legal definition of trafficking to conform with international requirements, ensure the appropriation of consistent resourcing for the anti-trafficking unit, and conduct sensitivity training to reduce victim blaming and breaches of victim confidentiality. (U.S. Department of State, 2005)

Such goals, however, seem far from realizable, given that Ukraine, for lack of funds and practical steps, is not yet even meeting its own less lofty goals. There are substantial gaps in the Comprehensive Program that have not yet been systematically addressed by those making recommendations for improvements. Nor have numerous critical issues yet been identified, discussed, and debated, in order for there to be real progress in meeting policy objectives, such as the link between violence against women in Ukraine and trafficking. It has been reported, for instance, that 50% of adult women in Ukraine have experienced violence (Rudd, 2002). The extent to which women seek employment abroad to escape oppressive and violent situations is still not fully understood.

Another overlooked issue is the public perception of trafficking, which is intimately related to sexism. As one researcher was told by police, government officials, and academic experts, "the reason so many women were being trafficked from Ukraine is because Ukraine has the most beautiful women in the world" (Hughes, 2005, p. 2). Commenting on her experiences as a field researcher, Hughes (2005) concluded that "at the end of these conversations and interviews I was often wondering whether I was studying sexism or trafficking" (p. 3). The public's attitude towards trafficking plays an unfavorable role. Many Ukrainians are certain that women who go abroad in search of jobs are mostly prostitutes and should not complain about their eventual circumstances. These kinds of responses underscore the extent to which the gendered dimensions of trafficking are obscured but fundamental. As Morrison (2005) correctly noted, "Gender cannot be separated from trafficking because gender discrimination is a key root cause that causes women to be trafficked from Ukraine."

Rethinking foundational categories of femininity and masculinity is critical to addressing the commodification of women's sexuality, now normalized and taken as a given, rather than a social and political construct. However, attention to gender relations should not be limited to the Ukrainian context. Approaches to the problem of trafficking must also address "the politics of gender in both sending and receiving countries" (Uehling, 2004, p. 86). In doing so, any full analysis also needs to consider the broader structural conditions created by globalization, which underpin all aspects of human trafficking, especially gender inequalities, since global problems such as trafficking "are those that by their very nature transcend the capacity of the nation-state to deal with them effectively as an independent entity" (von Struensee, 2000, p. 16). The full effects of globalization—from creating the ideal conditions for trafficking to flourish, to shaping the ways in which trafficking is understood, to allowing foreign influence to frame current notions and responses to the phenomenon—need to be revealed and interrogated.

GLOBALIZATION

Globalization can be understood as "a process by which nations, businesses, and people are becoming more connected and interdependent across the globe through increased economic integration, and communication exchange, cultural diffusion—especially of Western culture and travel" (Labonte & Torgerson, 2004, n.p.). Although not a new phenomenon, characteristics of the current wave include increasing global economic integration; the proliferation of multilateral agreements and related shifts in domestic policy; changing modes of production and patterns of consumption; population mobility and urbanization; cultural diffusion (especially Westernization); and technological advances (Maclean & Sicchia, 2004). Recent writing has clarified the wide-ranging impacts of globalization through different dimensions (such as Appaduria, 1990; Drager, Labonte, & Torgerson, 2002; Woodward, Drager, Beaglehole, & Lipson, 2001). However, more attention is required in order to illuminate the connections between economic globalization, disproportionately gendered effects of economic restructuring, changing gender roles in receiving and sending countries related to economic integration, and growing demand for sex-related service sectors (Gülçür & İlkkaracan, 2002). While some scholars argue that globalization is bringing about the downfall of patriarchy as a system of social organization, arguably, it has further entrenched inequality. In fact, globally "Women are disproportionately affected by poverty and limited economic options globally, and in postsocialist countries, this has also proven true" (Kligman & Limoncelli, 2005, p. 128).

The Commodification of Women's Labor and Bodies
Economic globalization has also given rise to the deeper commodification of women's labor and bodies, largely affecting life choices and chances. Nonetheless, debates continue over whether women who are trafficked have agency. For example, Doezema (2000) argued that "insisting on viewing these women as victims means denying that they can have agency in their own lives" (p. 35). Seeing trafficked women as total victims, Bruckert and Parent (2002) argued, "gives the victims no voice to explain the meaning of their actions and greatly reduces the scope of the problem of trafficking in humans" (p. 12). Similarly, as Gülçür and İlkkaracan (2002) explained, "although they are vulnerable to violence and discrimination, some migrant sex workers are paradoxically in control of their bodies and create their own survival mechanisms in a patriarchal world" (p. 418).

    At the same time, agency and consent are contentious. As Oxman-Martinez, Martinez, and Hanley (2005) argued, "when individuals 'choose' to be trafficked as a result of economic, political, or family pressures at home…this does not negate the fact that their human rights are being violated" (p. 15). Moreover, one must not lose sight of the fact that poverty is a key factor in women's increasing willingness to go abroad to seek work, thereby risking a trafficking situation (Rudd,

2002). Often, globalization creates the conditions for international employment opportunities without providing adequate protection for those women who leave their homes seeking a better economic future. The international community needs to consider the broader structural conditions that drive potential victims to look for ways out of their predicament and, indeed, to put themselves at risk for commodification (Oxman-Martinez, Martinez, & Hanley, 2001).

The International Demand for Sex Work
Related to this consideration is the need to explore the increased demand for sex trafficking. The very raison d'être of this phenomenon is the "export" of young women and girls for further exploitation in the sex industries of foreign countries (Lakiza-Sachuk, 2003). Ironically, many countries that have been at the forefront of critiquing Ukraine's policies and programs (including, but not limited to, the United States and Canada) are also important destination countries for women trafficked from Ukraine. Furthermore, destination countries often have laws and policies that enable and legitimize sex industries (Hughes & Denisova, 2001) and undermine efforts to work across borders to combat human trafficking.

In essence, sex trafficking sexualizes inequities between countries (Agathangelou & Ling, 2003). Destination countries are complicit in the "globalization of desire industries, like sex trafficking" (Agathangelou & Ling, 2003, p. 139) because they do not identify and address "the conditions of vulnerability that create a climate that fosters trafficking" (Clark, 2003, p. 260). Instead, they actually create that climate. The demand side of trafficking, however, is not prioritized in the efforts to halt it. As Hughes (2001) argued, "less attention is focused on curtailing demand" (p. 14). In a similar vein, Kligman and Limoncelli (2001) have argued that "Unless attention is focused on the demand side of trafficking—in all its forms—and poverty is not a resource for profit-driven entrepreneurs the world over, trafficking will continue not only to exist but to expand" (p. 131). Evidently, much more attention needs to be paid to the relationship between economic globalization and commodification that leads to the exploitation of the most vulnerable and to the profit and pleasure of those who benefit from trafficking. At the heart of this is the need for greater intergovernmental cooperation between origin and destination countries, in order for effective legal and medical responses to trafficking to be realized.

External Influences on Ukraine's Response to Trafficking, Including the Hegemony of Human-Rights Discourses
Funding of various domestically run programs, initiatives, and NGOs in Ukraine often comes from international donors. Influence, of course, lands with those foreign dollars. According to Hughes and Denisova (2001), "in setting their policies on...trafficking, these well-funded NGOs do not consult Ukrainian women or citizens in general, but adopt the position of their funders" and, as a corollary, "many grassroots NGOs that represent...views of the citizens...do not have the resources and access to conferences and policy forums that destination countries give the NGOs that represent their views" (pp. 19–20). Not only does this undermine local capacities vis-à-vis trafficking, it also undermines bottom-up efforts to determine and develop the most appropriate and effective *Ukrainian* responses to the problem. Accordingly, the authors of the report prepared by UNICEF, the OSCE, USAID, and the British Council have concluded that "however important international initiatives are, there is no doubt that the Government of Ukraine needs to be the main driving force behind coordinating in-country initiatives" (Lutsenko et al., 2005, p. 141).

The authentic voices of citizens in sending countries like Ukraine have thus "been supplanted by the voice of the destination countries, resulting in a corruption of civil society" (Hughes & Denisova, 2001, p. 5). As more foreign "help" and accompanying visions arrive, a certain framing of trafficking is becoming firmly ingrained. For instance, the current non-governmental sector is heavily invested in promoting the human rights of victims and working to foster the inclusion of trafficked women's rights in international instruments and national legislation. While rights discourse should inform the issue of sex trafficking and the rights of victims should be protected and promoted, this framing has become so entrenched that there is little recognition of the problem as possibly more than a rights issue; awareness of the gendered health dimensions of globalized sex trafficking is overshadowed.

Globalization, Trafficking, and Health
During the last decade, there has been growing interest in the effects of globalization on human health (see Cornia, 2001; Dollar, 2001; Doyal, 2004; Drager & Beaglehole, 2001; Harris & Seid, 2004). Research connecting globalization, gender, and health is only beginning to emerge (Hankivsky & Morrow, 2004; Maclean & Sicchia, 2004; Labonte & Torgenson, 2004). For example, in their recent edited collection, Maclean and Sicchia (2004, p. 8) investigated a diverse range of issues at the intersection of globalization, gender, and health, concluding that many existing analyses and empirical studies that explore linkages between gender and health fail to recognize gendered impacts. In addition, they identified food security, nutritional well-being, HIV/AIDS, tobacco, occupational health, mental health, infectious disease, violence, and reproductive health as priority health issues for more research, better measurement, and further documentation. The trafficking of women and its health impacts has also been identified as a key priority area for public health research (Maclean & Sicchia, 2004).

The health effects—in particular the mental health effects—of sexual trafficking on girls and women involved in the sex trade are similar to those documented in violence against women. According to preliminary research, trafficked women experience a range of physical and psychological health problems, including food and sleep deprivation; repeated rape; physical injury such as bruising, broken bones or teeth, mouth injuries, cuts, and burns; emotional manipulation including threats and blackmail; persistent sexual exploitation; social marginalization; sexually transmitted diseases, including HIV, and unwanted pregnancies from unsafe sexual practices such as condom refusal; forced or unsafe abortions, absence of gynecologic care and HIV testing; anxiety, substance misuse, depression, suicidality, somatized symptoms and other sequelae of abuse (such as headaches, body aches, dizziness, and nausea); and an inability to recuperate and integrate into society (Busza, Castle, & Diarra, 2004; Pisklakova & Sinelkinov, 2002; Stewart & Gajic-Veljanoski, 2005). Most trafficked persons suffer from post-traumatic stress disorder and, because of constant physical and psychological abuse, exhibit symptoms associated with survivors of severe trauma and torture (Pisklakova & Sinelnikov, 2002). However, while these consequences are slowly being recognized, the health effects of sex trafficking have not been prioritized in Ukraine's responses to date.

The cost of not adequately framing trafficking as a health issue is increased due to the fundamental weaknesses of the health care system in Ukraine, which has not been particularly effective in the areas of health education and promotion. Women lack information crucial to their health and to the health of their families, particularly in the areas of nutrition and breast feeding, family planning and the prevention of unwanted pregnancy, self-care during pregnancy, and the prevention of female cancers and other health problems. Services for STDs are not integrated into the general range of services. Violence against women is not addressed by the health sector in any systematic way. Women's preventive health care education, and health issues in general, are not being addressed with priority. With regard to the victims of trafficking, reports indicate that programs and services that could attend to their myriad health needs, including long-term psychological support, are not provided under the current assistance programs of either state agencies or NGOs (Lutsenko et al., 2005). Medical practitioners remain uninformed about the needs of trafficked women and have not developed appropriate treatment plans. Moreover, due to the lack of money in the health care system more generally, medical assistance is contingent on financial resources. As the 2005 report on trafficking in Ukraine indicated, "the quality of care given to any victim will be proportional to the amount of money in her pocket" (Lutsenko et al., p. 130). Furthermore, those who have attempted to work with state medical facilities to improve health-care-system responses to trafficking survivors report widespread financial corruption during the process of treating these vulnerable persons.

Rethinking Globalization, Human Rights, and Trafficking
Another serious implication of seeing human rights as a panacea to global injustices such as sex trafficking is that it undermines the search for an alternative social contract, a new ethics for a global order in which globalization is rethought, and trafficking is not only seen as a violation of human rights, but as a problem that undermines human health, itself a public good that is necessary for life to flourish. While scholars have started to explore alternative theoretical foundations to deal with the current challenges and deficits associated with globalization (Hankivsky, 2006; Singer, 2002), this work has not yet led to the development of "globalization with a human face" (UNDP, 1999). Moreover, universal human rights continue to be seen as the most effective way to protect against all forms of oppression and discrimination, even though they have also contributed to the creation of the global culture of neglect (Robinson, 1999). Indeed, trafficking coexists with strong international human-rights discourse.

What is required is a broadening of ethical and moral worldviews such that destructive and exploitative forces associated with globalization can be identified, problematized, and better responded to (Hankivsky, 2006, p. 97). In a globalized context, persons are not equally situated or empowered. As I have argued elsewhere, human beings have a range of needs that correspond to their particular situations at both the national and global levels, and they have different capacities and abilities to attend to their own needs (Hankivsky, 2005, p. 96). The explicit recognition of such realities would not only isolate the ways in which globalization creates the conditions that support trafficking but also create an opportunity to broaden the conceptualization of trafficking and to place health risks and consequences at the top of the agenda. Trafficking should not only be seen as a violation of human rights, but as an experience that fundamentally affects human health and well-being, as well undermines the ability of the most vulnerable and marginalized women to live the best possible lives they can.

CONCLUSION

Ukraine, which is considered the single largest country of origin for sex trafficking (Clark, 2003), is an ideal case study to scrutinize the forces that bear on any country's framing of human trafficking and prevention initiatives. This chapter has pointed to a number of shortcomings in Ukraine's internal antitrafficking programs. However, the discussion also highlights a largely uninvestigated dimension: the extent to which trafficking is a manifestation of globalization and, specifically, the role of the international community in shaping the conditions necessary for trafficking, and negatively influencing conceptualizations and responses to the problem. Reframing sex trafficking cannot only happen in origin countries like Ukraine. It is a challenge that belongs to the entire international community. Knowledge of the political, economic, and social contexts that enable trafficking, information about its profound impact on the health and well-being of women, and alternative visions for globalization are essential to rethinking the phenomenon of human trafficking and the realization of truly effective structural changes and interventions.

REFERENCES

Agathangelou, A., & Ling, L. (2003). Desire industries: Sex trafficking, UN peacekeeping, and the neo-liberal world order. *Brown Journal of World Affairs, 10*(1), 133–148.

Appadurai, A. (1990). Disjuncture and difference in the global cultural economy. *Theory, Culture, and Society, 7,* 295–310.

Bruckert, C., & Parent, C. (2002). *Trafficking in human beings and organized crime: A literature review.* RCMP Research and Evaluation Branch, Community, Contract and Aboriginal Policing Service Directorate. Retrieved January 23, 2007, from http://www.rcmp-grc.gc.ca/ccaps/traffick_e.htm

Busza, J., Castle, S., & Diarra, A. (2004). Trafficking and health. *British Medical Journal, 328,* 1369–1371.

Clark, M. (2003). Human trafficking casts shadow on globalization. *YaleGlobal, 23.* Retrieved December 16, 2006, from http://yaleglobal.yale.edu/display.article?id=1448

Cornia, G. (2001). Globalization and health: Results and options. *Bulletin of the World Health Organization, 79*(9), 834–841.

Doezema, J. (2000). Loose women or lost women? The re-emergence of the myth of 'white slavery' in contemporary discourses of trafficking in women. *Gender Issues, 18*(1), 23–50.

Dollar, D. (2001). Is globalization good for your health? *Bulletin of the World Health Organization, 79*(9), 180.

Doyal, L. (2004). Women, health and global restructuring: Setting the scene. *Development, 47*(2), 18–23.

Drager, N., & Beaglehole, R. (2001). Globalization: Changing the public health landscape. Editorial. *Bulletin of the World Health Organization, 79,* 803.

Drager, N., Labonte, R., & Torgenson, R. (2002). *Frameworks for analyzing the links between globalization and health.* Draft document. Retrieved January 21, 2007, from http://www.ukglobalhealth. org/content/Text/Analytical_Framework_Paper.pdf

Emke-Poulopoulos, I. (2001). *Migrant trafficking and prostitution in Greece.* (Working Paper No. 2). Athens, Greece: Panteion University, Mediterranean Migration Observatory, Urban Environment and Human Resources Research Institute.

Gülçür, L., & İlkkaracan, P. (2002). The "Natasha" experience: Migrant sex workers from the former Soviet Union and Eastern Europe in Turkey. *Women's Studies International Forum, 25*(4), 411–421.

Hankivsky, O. (2005). *Social policy and the ethic of care.* Vancouver, Canada: University of British Columbia Press.

Hankivsky, O. (2006). Imagining ethical globalization. *Journal of Global Ethics, 2*(1), 91–110.

Hankivsky, O., & Morrow, M. (2004). *Trade agreements, home care and women's health.* Ottawa, Canada: Status of Women Canada.

Hankivsky, O., Morrow, M., & Varcoe, C. (2004). Women and violence: The effects of dismantling the welfare state. *Critical Social Policy, 24*(3), 358–384.

Harris, R., & Seid, M. (2004). Globalization and health in the new millennium. In R. Harris & M. Seid, (Eds.), *Globalization and Health* (pp. 1–46). Amsterdam: Brill.

Hughes, D. (2001). The "Natasha" trade: Transnational sex trafficking. *National Institute of Justice Journal, 246,* 9–15.

Hughes, D. (2005, March 5). *Combating sex trafficking: Advancing freedom for women and girls.* Keynote address For the Northeast Women's Studies Association Annual Conference at University of Massachusetts, Dartmouth, MA. Retrieved December 29, 2006, from http:// www.uri.edu/artsci/wms/hughes/combating_sex_trafficking.doc

Hughes, D., & Denisova, T. (2001). The transnational political criminal nexus of trafficking in women from Ukraine. *Trends in Organized Crime, 6*(3/4), 1–22.

Human Rights Watch Europe and Asia Division. (2003). Women's work: Discrimination against women in the Ukrainian labor force (Research report). *Human Rights Watch, 15*(5D). Retrieved March 3, 2008, from http://www.hrw.org/reports/2003/ukraine0803/

IOM (International Organization for Migration). (1995, May). *Trafficking and prostitution: The growing exploitation of migrant women from Central and Eastern Europe* (Study conducted by the IOM Migration Information Program). Geneva, Switzerland: Author.

IOM (International Organization for Migration). (2001, April). New IOM figures on the global scale of trafficking. *Trafficking in Migrants Quarterly Bulletin, 23.*

Kligman, G., & Limoncelli, S. (2005). Trafficking women after socialism: To, through, and from Eastern Europe. *Social Politics, 12*(1), 118–140.

Labonte, R., & Torgerson, R. (2004). Globalization and health (Portion of online research report; H. Maclean, S. Sicchia, & R. Labonte, Eds.). Prepared for the Institute of Gender and Health, Canadian Institutes of Health Research, Ottawa, Canada. Retrieved March 3, 2008, from http://www.womensresearch.ca/news/reports.php

Lakiza-Sachuk, N. (2003). *Trafficking in women from Ukraine as a security issue. Conference presentation.* Washington, DC: Publication of the Transnational Crime and Corruption Center.

Lazaridis, G. (2001). Trafficking and prostitution: The growing exploitation of migrant women in Greece. *European Journal of Women's Studies, 8,* 67–102.

Lutsenko, Y., Matiaszek, L., Scanlan, S., Shab., I. (2005). *Trafficking in Ukraine: An assessment of current responses* (Multiparty research report). Kiev, Ukraine: UNICEF, Organization for Security and Cooperation in Europe (OSCE), USAID, and the British Council. Retrieved March 3, 2008, from http://www.unicef.org/ukraine/trafficking(1).pdf

Maclean, H., & Sicchia, S. (2004, April 27). *Gender, globalization and health: Excerpts from the background paper.* Paper presented at the NIH Stone House Forum, Bethesda, MD. Retrieved February 2, 2007, from http://www.crwh.org/PDF/Stonehouse-Abridged.pdf

Miko, F., & Park, G. (2003, May 10). *Report for Congress. Trafficking in women and children: The U.S. and international response* (Congressional Research Service Report 98-649 C).

Morrison, L. (2003). *Trafficking and Ukraine lesson plan.* Ukraine.

Peace Corps, Washington, DC. (n.d.). Retrieved February 2, 2007, from http://pcukraine.org/members/lessons/686_2.doc

Oxman-Martinez, J., Martinez, A., & Hanley, J. (2001). Human trafficking: Canadian government policy and practice. *Refuge, 19*(4), 14–23.

Pisklakova, M., & Sinelnikov, A. (2002). What dreams may become: Trafficked women and their resultant health issues. *Common Health, 10*(10), 64–68.

Pyshchulina, O. (2005). An evaluation of Ukrainian legislation to counter and criminalize human trafficking. In S. Stoecker & L. Shelley (Eds.), *Human trafficking and transnational crime: Eurasian and American perspectives* (pp. 115–124). London: Rowman & Littlefield Publishers.

Rasner, M. (2004, December 9). Ukraine's top dissident raises a rare female voice. *Women's News.* Retrieved December 16, 2006, from http://www.womensenews.org/article.cfm/dyn/aid/2101/context/archive

RISU (Religious Information Service of Ukraine). (2005). *Government asks churches to help victims of slave trade.* Retrieved January 21, 2007, from http://www.risu.org.ua/eng/news/article; 7376

Robinson, F. (1999). *Globalizing care: Ethics, feminist theory, and international relations.* Boulder, CO: Westview Press.

Rudd, J. (2002). *Summary report of trafficking of women in Ukraine* (Research report). Winrock International and the U.S. Agency for International Development. Retrieved December 16, 2006, from http://www.winrock.org/leadership/files/SummaryTrafficUkraine. pdf#search=%22Rudd%2C%20J.%202002.%20Summary%20Report %20of%20Trafficking%20of%20Women%20in%20Ukraine%22

Singer, J. (2003). *The world of human trafficking: An unacceptable violation of human rights.* London: National Missing Persons Helpline.

Stewart, D., & Gajic-Veljanoski, O. (2005). Trafficking in women: the Canadian perspective. *Canadian Medical Association Journals, 173*(1), 25–26.

Time International. (2001). Human slavery: Eastern Europe has become the fastest-growing point of origin for the trafficking of females for sex. Law enforcement has been slow to respond. *Time International, 157*(7), 18.

Uehling, G. (2004). Irregular and illegal migration through Ukraine. *International Migration, 42*(3), 77–109.

UNDP (United Nations Development Programme). (1999). *Human development report 1999.* New York: Oxford University Press.

UNICEF. (2001). *Profiting from abuse.* New York: United Nations Children's Fund.

United Nations. (2000). *Convention against transnational organized crime, annex II: Protocol to prevent, suppress and punish trafficking in persons, especially women and children. A/55/383. Article 3.* New York: Author.

U.S. Department of State. (2005, June 3). Remarks by Secretary of State Condoleezza Rice on the release of the 5th annual Department of State *Trafficking in Persons Report.* Washington, DC. Retrieved December 16, 2006, from http://www.state.gov/secretary/rm/2005/47193.htm

U.S. Department of State. (2007, June 12). *Victims of Trafficking and Violence Protection Act of 2000: Trafficking in persons report 2007.* Washington, DC: Author. Retrieved March 4, 2008, from http://www.state.gov/g/tip/rls/tiprpt/2007/

von Struensee, V. (2000). Globalized, wired, sex trafficking in women and children. *Murdoch University Electronic Journal of Law, 7*(2), 1–69.

Winrock International. (2001). *Nationwide survey: Trafficking women as a social problem in Ukrainian society, summary findings* (Research survey). Kyiv, Ukraine: The Social Monitoring Center and the Ukrainian Institute of Social Studies. Retrieved December 30, 2006, from http://www.winrock.org/leadership/files/SocialMonitoring.pdf

Woodward, D., Drager, N., Beaglehole, R., & Lipson, D. (2001). Globalization and health: A framework for analysis and action. *Bulletin of the World Health Organization, 79*(9), 875–881.

ENDNOTE

1. The information and lobby campaigns focus on providing expertise on legislative acts regarding the status of women in Ukraine, conducting roundtable discussions on the problem, and cooperating with national and international government and nongovernment organizations in Ukraine and abroad in order to prevent trafficking in persons. The prevention-education campaign involves conducting educational activities among youth, training trainers, and publishing information materials and guidelines. The social-assistance campaign organizes medical, psychological, and legal assistance for trafficking victims and conducts roundtable discussions with other stakeholders in social services. The hotline is a service available for consulting and assisting trafficking victims directly; consulting with women who are going to work, study, or marry abroad; and for collecting data.

CHAPTER 8

ROUTINE HIV TESTING OF WOMEN IN HIGH-PREVALENCE AREAS:

A PROBLEM OF STIGMA, DISCRIMINATION, AND VIOLENCE

Heather Worth

The consequences of HIV antibody testing differ from those of many other tests that are used in medicine today. This test can seriously harm persons being tested, the communities to which they belong and society as a whole. At the same time, there are many great benefits to be obtained from its use. This test, in raising many complex dilemmas and issues, is symbolic of the many problems that we are being faced with by the HIV epidemic…Consequently, great caution is needed in deciding how we, as a society, will govern that use.

—Bayer (1989, p. 119)

INTRODUCTION

On the Saturday before the 2004 International AIDS Conference in Bangkok, a new joint United Nations Program on HIV/AIDS (UNAIDS) and a World Health Organization (WHO) policy statement on routine HIV testing in high-prevalence countries was issued and released to the international media. It argued that the numbers of people in low- and medium-income countries who are taking HIV tests was low and, as anti-retroviral treatment (ART) is scaled up, there was a need to dramatically increase the numbers of people testing: "To reach people in need of treatment, tens of millions of tests will have to be conducted among those who may have been exposed to HIV" (UNAIDS/WHO, 2004, p. 1).

The initiative that captured the spirit of that statement, called "3 by 5" (targeting 3 million people by 2005), has now been replaced with a new initiative, "Universal Access to HIV/AIDS Prevention, Care and Treatment," which still has at its core provider-initiated testing—a stepped-up approach to testing in which health providers routinely test for HIV in clinical settings unless a patient actively opts out of testing and counseling. As Ron Bayer (1989) argued, testing tens of millions of people for HIV in the resource-poor world brings to the fore complex issues and dilemmas. Of particular concern is the impact of provider-initiated testing on women, which is based on a highly problematic ideal of "success," measured in terms of numbers of tests and, at best, a speculative link between the numbers of women tested and the numbers on ART.

From the beginning, the HIV pandemic has been accompanied by widespread fear, stigma, discrimination, and violence against those who are HIV-positive or are held to be the vectors of infection. Women who are infected with HIV generally have a lack of economic, social, and sexual power, so it is no wonder that they have faced much of the blame for the virus' spread. The particular inequities women face in the HIV pandemic have been well documented (as shall be described later). This chapter examines some of the gendered problematics of the new policy rollout on routine HIV testing in high-prevalence countries, with the aim of going beyond the numbers to analyze the social and cultural impact of routine testing not only on the lives of those women testing positive, but also on the lives of those testing negative.

"3 BY 5," "UNIVERSAL ACCESS," AND PROVIDER-INITIATED ROUTINE HIV TESTING

"The current strategy—in which patients specifically request an HIV test—is not working in developing countries, where 90% of HIV-positive people do not know their statuses, U.N. officials said" (Ross, 2004).

The "3 by 5" program and its successor, "Universal Access to HIV/AIDS Prevention, Care and Treatment," are responses to the obviously inequitable global distribution of ART, the realization that morbidity and mortality consequent from HIV infection will further impoverish nations through a decline in production, and that there will be a drop in expenditure on education in those places combined with skewed expenditure on health—in fact, it was clear HIV would be an accelerator of the very socioeconomic and political forces which ensured its uneven spread in the first place.

The goal of the "3 by 5" program was to deliver ART to 3 million people in low- and middle-income countries by 2005. According to WHO/UNAIDS officials, in order to achieve this, HIV testing would need to be dramatically scaled up. As the first WHO/UNAIDS (2004) "3 by 5" progress report stated,

> Identifying 3 million people needing treatment requires identifying 20 million people living with HIV, assuming that 15% need treatment at any one time. If the overall HIV prevalence across the focus countries is 10%, *200 million people would need to be tested* [italics added] to identify the 20 million with HIV. (WHO/UNAIDS, 2004, p. 27)[1]

People in high-prevalence countries have been slow to take up HIV testing for a number of reasons. These include the lack of availability of both ART and HIV testing programs, which is a consequence of the interrelated problems of inadequate health-care-service infrastructure and a dearth of human resources (see WHO/UNAIDS, 2004, p. 4). Moreover, many are still unaware of the benefits of ART, and there are cultural constraints on using testing programs and other Western developed medical procedures and drugs such as ART (Office of the Special Advisor for Africa [OSAA], 2004–2005, p. 4). Most importantly, however, is the issue that this chapter addresses; namely, that many people, particularly women, face very real issues of violence, personal abandonment, and shunning by the community resulting from a positive HIV-test result, consequences that may not be assuaged by ART (see, e.g., Maman, Mbwambo, Hogan, & Kilonzo, 2002). For many women in resource-constrained settings, an HIV-positive test is still equated with having to face death.

The possibility of financing a global rollout of ART via the new Global Fund to Fight AIDS, Tuberculosis, and Malaria and other large donor organization programs generated a groundswell of calls for provider-initiated, "opt out," routine HIV testing. A report of a WHO consultation that took place in November 2002 indicated that, given the still-growing crisis in the epidemic, and the funding now available, new approaches to HIV testing needed implementing to "mov[e] beyond the model of provision that relies entirely upon individuals seeking out help for themselves to permit broader access for all. In this new approach, such services will become a routine part of health care" (World Health Organization [WHO], 2003, p. 3). Added to this, there have been other calls (mostly by the United States) for a change in approach to HIV testing. According to the president's Emergency Plan for AIDS Relief (Office of the United States Global AIDS Coordinator) report released in February 2004, a key priority is to implement "good policies," which include "encouraging the adoption of routine testing policies" (p. 30). In a 2002 Lancet article, De Cock, Marum, and Mbori-Ngacha argued that

> we think that Africa would now benefit most from an approach to HIV/AIDS based on a public health model that includes voluntary counselling, testing, and partner notification; routine HIV testing in prevention services such as prevention of mother-to-child transmission, and treatment for sexually transmitted infections; routine

diagnostic HIV testing for patients seeking medical treatment (e.g., for tuberculosis); and enhanced access to HIV/AIDS care. (p. 69)

The United States-based Global Business Coalition on HIV/AIDS (GBC) also held strong opinions on the subject as illustrated in a press article by the president of the GBC, Richard Holbrooke (who is also former U.S. ambassador to the United Nations), and Richard Furman, a thoracic surgeon, who is a founder of World Medical Mission: "No amount of money…will be enough to bring the disease under control until we focus on testing, the missing front in the battle against AIDS" (Holbrooke & Furman, 2004, p. A25). As they put it, "It is time to abandon this ethnocentric Western rhetoric, born in the 1980's in the United States under different circumstances, that led to the 'V for voluntary' in Voluntary Counseling and Testing" (p. A25). Neither of these articles raised the question of violence against women as a consequence of large-scale routinized testing. Furthermore, at a Geneva meeting in February 2004, members of the WHO Global TB/HIV Core Group "pleaded strongly for much more assertive action in promoting HIV diagnostic testing in patients seeking medical care, in combination with a 'serostatus' public health approach in the general population" (WHO TB/HIV Working Group, 2004, p. 2).

In July 2004 a joint UNAIDS/WHO policy statement was issued, which stated that HIV testing and counseling was paramount in treatment (and in prevention), but that only 10% of those who needed testing had access to it. It went on to argue that when a patient presents with symptoms, not only voluntary counseling and testing (VCT) should be encouraged, but also diagnostic HIV testing, and that such efforts needed to go even further:

> A **routine offer of HIV testing by health care providers** should be made to all patients being:
>
> • assessed in a **sexually transmitted infection** clinic or elsewhere for a sexually transmitted infection—to facilitate tailored counselling based on knowledge of HIV status

- seen in the context of pregnancy—to facilitate an offer of **antiretroviral prevention of mother-to-child transmission**
- seen in clinical and community based health service settings where **HIV is prevalent and antiretroviral treatment is available** (injecting drug use treatment services, hospital emergencies, internal medicine hospital wards, consultations etc.) but who are **asymptomatic** [bold in original] (UNAIDS/WHO, 2004, p. 2)

The move to provider-initiated, routine (opt out) HIV testing has a number of underlying gendered assumptions, and makes a number of claims about the efficacy of this approach compared with voluntary counseling and testing. Some of these are that voluntary testing has failed in women; a human-rights approach to HIV prevention is wrong for resource-poor countries; routine testing not only accelerates HIV-prevention programs but is in itself an effective HIV-prevention mechanism for women; and HIV testing and the concomitant rollout of ART reduce stigma and discrimination against women.

The "3 by 5" program ended in December 2005 with the likelihood of a large increase in the number of people tested (although global data are not currently available, particularly those that show testing by gender). The WHO/UNAIDS report (2006) showed that, for example, the scaling up of a routine offer of testing in clinics across Botswana produced an increase in the percentage of pregnant women receiving testing and counseling between March 2004 and December 2005, and "Botswana now estimates that 25% of its population of 1.7 million now know their HIV status" (WHO/UNAIDS, 2006, p. 54). However, numbers of tests carried out in Botswana health care clinics is not necessarily an indicator of the success of provider-initiated testing. There is new evidence from Botswana that while the introduction of routine testing has meant an increase in the number of pregnant women being tested, there has not been a concomitant increase in those returning to receive their test results (Seipone et al., 2004). This may mean that routine testing is being carried out without women being able to opt out.

In general, however, there is a lack of data documenting any negative consequences arising from the initiative, and a paucity of findings on the specific consequences of routine HIV testing on women. While the important documents of the "3 by 5" and "Universal Access" initiatives do raise the problem of gender inequity, the major document launching the "3 by 5," entitled *Treating 3 Million by 2005, Making It Happen* (WHO/UNAIDS, 2003), mentions women only twice. The problem of stigma and discrimination faced by those women living with the virus, meanwhile, are glossed over. On page 6 of the document, the claim is made that universal access to ART

> opens up ways to accelerate prevention in communities in which people will know their status—and, critically, will **want** [bold in original] to know their status. As HIV/AIDS becomes a disease that can be both prevented and treated, attitudes will change, and denial, stigma and discrimination will rapidly be reduced. (WHO/ UNAIDS, 2003, p. 6)

However, there is a complete lack of information about *how* this ideal will be met, apart from rather circular references later in the document to reducing HIV/AIDS stigma and discrimination through ART programs (WHO/UNAIDS, 2003, pp. 17, 38, 50).

Similarly, the 2004 UNAIDS/WHO Policy on HIV testing does not specifically mention women. Rather, they are implied in the context of pregnancy (as mentioned previously). With regards to other issues, the document does state that

> The reality is that stigma and discrimination continue to stop people from having an HIV test. To address this, the cornerstones of HIV testing scale-up must include improved protection from stigma and discrimination as well as assured access to integrated prevention, treatment and care services. The conditions under which people undergo HIV testing must be anchored in a human rights approach which protects their human rights and pays due respect to ethical principles. (UNAIDS/WHO, 2004, p. 1)

Nonetheless, it is clear that despite the heartfelt intentions contained in these statements, they have little power in protecting many women who actually undergo testing. If we examine the final WHO/UNAIDS "3 by 5" report, the claims for this human rights-based approach seem rather less certain. Here, the authors admit that "[s]tigma and discrimination remain two of our most stubborn obstacles," but they go on to blame international donors and national funders, whose response "while ever more robust, has not been sufficient to meet this enormous challenge" (WHO/UNAIDS, 2006, p. 5). The report argued that in Lesotho, for example, too few people know their HIV status due to a "shortage of testing and counselling sites and stigma and fear associated with HIV...As a result, those who are already infected are likely to continue to infect others unknowingly and are not obtaining access to care and support" (p. 54).

This blame seems particularly misplaced, given that by its own account, the UN has had difficulty managing the huge amounts of confidential information that flow from provider-initiated testing. We catch a glimpse of the seriousness of the problem of confidentiality and HIV testing in the recent UN document on the new "Universal Access" initiative, which recognizes that in the "3 by 5" rollout,

> [i]nsufficient access to confidential HIV testing was cited in consultations in Albania, Bangladesh, Botswana, Cambodia, Ethiopia, Gabon, Papua New Guinea, the Republic of Moldova, Romania, Somalia, Suriname, the former Yugoslav Republic of Macedonia, Trinidad and Tobago and the United Nations-administered province of Kosovo. Some high burden countries reported that they now routinely offer HIV testing to patients in all clinical and community-based health-service settings. Greater resources and political commitment must be mobilized to address problems of stigma, discrimination, gender and human rights. (United Nations, 2006, p. 16)

The problem of gender inequality is one of the greatest problems facing women in the epidemic, and has been a major stumbling block in addressing all aspects of HIV prevention, treatment, and care across the globe.

Because of its centrality in social life, the outcome of inequity—stigma and discrimination—will not just wilt away because women accept an HIV test. Just as inequality, in general, has been a driver of the HIV epidemic and a major contributor to its impact, the new policy of routine HIV testing may further exacerbate the gender inequality, which has put women at increased risk of HIV in the first place.

GENDERED ASSUMPTIONS ABOUT PROVIDER-INITIATED ROUTINE (OPT OUT) HIV TESTING

> Wouldn't greater knowledge of one's status—held in the strictest confidence (an essential part of any testing program)—greatly modify behavior, both for those who are HIV-positive and for the large majority who, even in the worst hit areas, are not infected? And wouldn't the greatest beneficiaries be women, who are all too often helpless victims but who do not know either their own status or that of any man in their life—and who have no way of getting their men to be tested.
>
> —Holbrooke (2006, p. A17)

Since the beginning of the epidemic there has been documented evidence that women face extreme HIV-related stigma, discrimination, and violence. In the early years, most of the published literature examined women's experience in the resource-rich world (see, e.g., McNaughton, 1992; Pizzi, 1992; Shane & Kaplan, 1991). More recently, a plethora of studies have shown that women from low-income, high-prevalence countries face similar issues of shaming, violence, and abandonment (see, e.g., Chandra, Deepthivarma, & Manjula, 2003; de Bruyn & Paxton, 2005; Kalichman & Simbayi, 2004; Letamo, 2003; Mawar, Saha, Pandit, & Mahajan, 2005; Mill, 2003; Mwamburi, Dladla, Qwana, & Lurie, 2005; Nyblade & Field-Nguer, 2001; Pignatelli et al., 2006).

I will juxtapose this history of HIV-related violence against women with the justification of routine HIV testing of women in the context of an accelerated rollout of ART. Firstly, I want to discuss why even client-initiated testing of women may have failed. Holbrooke and Furman

(2004) stated that in their whistle-stop tour of Africa they "witnessed a terrible truth that no one wants to admit: almost no one actually gets tested" (p. A25). Some of the issues of nontesting are to do with expense and difficulties of implementation (WHO/UNAIDS, 2003, p. 10). Moreover, VCT is woefully unavailable in many parts of Africa, and as the 2002 WHO Consultation report stated, "widespread ignorance of HIV status is the direct result of people's poor access to HIV testing, or to serious problems with its delivery and uptake" (WHO, 2003, p. 3). However, this does not necessarily mean VCT is to blame, or that its replacement with provider-initiated testing will work more efficiently and effectively. It is rather the case, as Sofia Gruskin (2004) stated in her article in the *Canadian HIV/AIDS Policy and Law Review*, that VCT "has not been sufficiently emphasized in many national responses to AIDS" (p. 3). While De Cock, Marum, and Mbori-Ngacha (2003) argued that high awareness of HIV in Africa reduces the need for extensive pretest counseling (which prepares those testing for the possibility of an HIV-positive result), Muersing and Sibind's (2000) findings from their work in Zimbabwe demonstrated the importance of pretest and posttest counseling. They argued that "the complex and changing nature of clients' needs indicates that common short-cuts in counseling are seriously flawed as a strategy to prepare [HIV-positive] clients for coping," (p. 17), and that "pre- and post-test counseling should be seen as a beginning and a necessary minimum of services" (p. 22).

Recent evidence indicates that HIV-related violence of one sort or another has not abated in the period of increased response to the problem. Nyblade and Field-Nguer's (2001) research in Zambia and Botswana indicated that blame for bringing HIV into the relationship does occur if women test positive (p. 33). Maman et al.'s (2002) research showed that the primary barrier to women being tested was the fear of conflict with their partners. The meanings partners ascribe to being tested are important barriers in seeking testing: women in the study felt that testing could threaten the relationship; they felt little autonomy in making the decision to test; and they were frightened of their partner's reaction (Maman et al., 2002, pp. 14–15). Malawi health authorities have also reported that pregnant women in that country have been attacked by spouses and boyfriends when they go to be tested for HIV (BBC, 2006). What is the point of knowing your status when this may well lead to violence?

Of course, the major problem for a woman being tested for HIV is the pressure for her both to disclose her status to a male partner (whether it is HIV-positive or HIV-negative), and to change her behavior, an act that would involve her partner also changing his behavior. Many women are not in a position to initiate a request for their partner to use a condom, let alone explain the reason for such a request. Indeed, it is women's disclosure of status that seems to be the point at which most violence occurs. Maman et al. (2002) indicated that disclosure of status could lead to both verbal and physical violence. Findings from their study show that HIV-positive women were 2.68 times more likely than HIV-negative women to have been beaten by their current partner, a figure which rose to 10 times more likely for young women (18–29 years old). Nonetheless, HIV testing pushes women into the position of having to disclose their serostatus, or is seen as tantamount to disclosure (Burke, 2006).

There is a widespread belief that the introduction of ART will reduce stigma and discrimination (or perhaps more appropriately "structural violence"[2]) against women, and a large-scale rollout of the drugs will be an incentive to test for HIV, resulting in further decreases in stigma and discrimination.

> In providing HIV treatment, we can achieve many other things at the same time. For example, by increasing access to ART, we have learnt that we can reduce the stigma associated with HIV infection. In the first world, the availability of ART—which can dramatically transform dying people back into healthy, productive individuals—was a critical factor in reducing the stigma associated with HIV and in enabling people to resume their lives. (Kim, 2004, p. 1)

This logic is debatable, but there is some evidence that it is true. Walton, Farmer, Lambert, Le' Andre, Koenig, and Mukherjee's (2005) work has convincingly indicated that in Haiti there was "a sharp decline in

AIDS-related stigma since the introduction of HAART" (p. 54). In Haiti, however, there was not just a rollout of HIV testing (in Haiti testing is voluntary), but a comprehensive AIDS prevention program and improved medical care. Apart from Haiti, this has not widely been the case. As argued previously, there is little support for the contention that widespread availability of HIV testing in resource-poor settings has resulted in a decrease of intolerance towards women who tested positive.

In the absence of a wide-ranging and inclusive set of health-promotion activities, antidiscrimination programs, and proper health care, the reliance on the clinic to carry out routine testing in a situation where only 0.15% of the HIV-positive population (15% of the 10% found to be positive) are able to access ART may in fact exacerbate stigma, discrimination, and structural violence for those found to be HIV-positive. The targeted settings for routine testing are: TB services, antenatal and family planning clinics, STI clinics, and injecting drug use sites. These setting either spotlight the familiar "at-risk" groups (sex workers and junkies), or, as in the cases of antenatal clinics and family planning clinics, intentionally focus on women who are most vulnerable to stigma and discrimination.

Increasingly, there have been claims that a human-rights approach, which is intimately linked to voluntary, client-initiated, confidential testing, has not worked in resource-poor settings. For example, the late Jim Yong Kim, the former director of HIV/AIDS of the World Health Organization, claimed that the "World Health Organization has decided that access to lifesaving therapies outweighs the need to avoid potential discrimination" (cited in Ross, 2004, n.p.). Similarly, De Cock et al. (2002) have claimed that "making AIDS a human rights issue has not succeeded," and that "the emphasis on public health has reduced the importance of public health and social justice" (p. 68). However, this is to deny the experiences of women in the epidemic. The human rights of women who may risk injury, abandonment, or even death if they test HIV-positive are not an abstract concept but an absolute reality.

One of the major ideas of routine testing is to do away with pretest counseling while leaving in place some posttest counseling. In many places there has only been a very simplified form of pretest counseling (see WHO/UNAIDS, 2003, p. 44), which, as Crewe and Viljoen (2005) have stated, is, in practice, "an adapted, incomplete counseling session, consisting of minimal information, or a mere request (by the test provider) to be tested" (p. 7). However, what seems to be one of the militating factors in women successfully taking up testing for HIV is proper preparation for the possibility of a positive result and the steps women will need to take in order to protect themselves from violence (see Maman et al. 2002; Pignatelli 2006). Women need support in the pretest period—their most uncertain period, and the one in which they face up to the possible consequences that a positive test might bring. Moreover, Pignatelli et al. (2006) pointed to the need for mass education campaigns that address stigma and discrimination before the rollout of any kind of wide-scale testing, a proposition that has come too late for the "3 by 5" program but could nonetheless inflect policy directions from here on in. To date, however, it is the clinic as the place of testing and the individualization of the process of testing (even when it is widespread) that have had the greatest emphasis.

Human-rights concerns must be focused on the ability of women who find themselves in a situation of routine testing to say "no" to routine offers of testing or to give fully informed consent under these circumstances. But as Csete, Shleifer, and Cohen, (2004, p. 494) argued, AIDS-related human-rights concerns are intricately related to informed consent, but encompass more than just this; they also include unequal gender relations, stigma and discrimination, and the right to information and services. Until the response to HIV is grounded in the community and there are positive social changes in the lives of women that protect them from violence when they test for HIV, until "the health system is strengthened, and an end to discrimination against people who are HIV-positive, testing will not succeed" (Rubenstein, 2004).

One of the major claims about routine HIV testing is that it acts as a good HIV-prevention mechanism. In their controversial piece, "Shadow on the Continent," De Cock et al. (2002) argued that

> a stated goal for prevention should be for every citizen, including sexually active adolescents, to know their HIV status, and for

repeat testing to occur at regular intervals. This approach would demystify HIV/AIDS, place the responsibility for avoidance of acquiring or transmitting HIV on every individual, and empower the community to take charge of its own health. (p. 70)

However, the evidence that testing prevents HIV is not strong, even in resource-rich countries; not only is the support for this position scant and conflicting, but there is actually evidence that where testing *is* used as a prevention mechanism, its effect is deleterious because it may give a sense of invulnerability to those who test negative and, among men, may undermine condom use (Kippax, 2006). One of the most controversial aspects of HIV testing as a primary means of HIV prevention is that it places HIV prevention in the clinic aimed at individualized and privatized outside-of-community initiatives. Of course, it is women who most often attend health care clinics, particularly for antenatal care. It is in this context that routine testing has its most conspicuous gender dimension: women are more likely to present in health care settings for routine testing. In a nutshell, as Rennie and Behets (2005) indicated, it is probably "easier in the short term to increase the numbers of tested women than it will be to protect the growing numbers of HIV-positive women from gender-based violence" (p. 55).

CONCLUSION

Testing should be required at marriage, before childbirth and upon any visit to a hospital. At these moments (and we hope, others) public health criteria legitimately take priority over the desire of the individual. This has historically been the case with contagious diseases.

—Holbrooke and Furman (2004, p. A25)

While HIV-related violence against women was identified very early on in the epidemic, it still fades into the background in the drive to accelerate ART through the increased rollout of HIV testing. Delivering health care services fits a traditional public-health model, where indicators of success are measured in numbers of people treated. However, HIV is not a disease like most others. Routine HIV testing, when delivered in a traditional public-health mode, may be efficient and effective in terms of numbers tested, but it may very well fail to address the social change necessary to ensure that women are able to test with impunity. Routine testing may also further medicalize the epidemic by taking HIV prevention out of the community and responsibility away from the state, and then putting it back into the clinic (where it is targeted mostly at women) and (paradoxically) into individualized solutions (women alone taking the responsibility for halting the spread of HIV). At the same time, the approach to routine testing is compatible with a neoliberal approach to health where responsibility for HIV testing lies with the individual woman who can make rational choices about her life and her health. Naturally, in this approach, the problem of men being as central to the spread of the pandemic as women, and as hard hit by its impact, is left unanalyzed, as is the problem of unequal relations between men and women that lies at the heart of much of the epidemic.

As this chapter was being finalized, the WHO evaluation of the "3 by 5" project was released. The issues which I have raised here are not addressed at all in the evaluation document, although there is a comment to the effect that

> ICW [the International Community of Women Living with AIDS] felt that gender issues relevant to HIV and AIDS were initially ignored in "3 by 5," but that the situation is now improving, with the importance of including gender issues becoming better understood. (Nemes et al., 2006, p. 77)

Further work analyzing the gaps and silences in that document is now needed.

The call for routine HIV testing assumes that it solves the problems associated with client-initiated testing of women, that women no longer need human rights to ensure their safety and protection, that accelerated testing will reduce the HIV-related stigma and violence women face on a daily basis, and that the consequent rollout of ARTs will assure women of a positive future. In fact, routine HIV testing will not solve the profound dislocation experienced by women who are diagnosed HIV-positive, nor the continued attempts to blame women in general for the spread of the virus. Making HIV a clinic-based, routinized part of health care, particularly in the antenatal setting, exacerbates the view of women as solely being child-bearers, and therefore having fewer rights in their own person. Moreover, knowledge of HIV status cannot produce changes in sexual practice in the context of highly gendered and unequal sexual relationships. Stigma and discrimination against women are central hindrances to the fight against HIV, not an adjunct to the acceleration of routine testing. We absolutely need to scale up ART, but not at the expense of women's lives.

REFERENCES

Bayer, R. (1989). Ethical and social policy issues raised by HIV screening: The epidemic evolves and so do the challenges. *AIDS, 3,* 119–124.

BBC. (2006). *Mums-to-be shun Malawi HIV tests.* BBC News Report. Retrieved March 31, 2007, from http://news.bbc.co.uk/2/hi/africa/4551767.stm

de Bruyn, M., & Paxton, S. (2005). HIV testing of pregnant women— What is needed to protect positive women's needs and rights? *Sexual Health, 2*(3), 143–151.

Burke, M. (2006, May). *Male factors influencing participation in PMTCT programs in Tanzania.* Paper presented at the Australian Federation of AIDS Organisations (AFAO) HIV Educators Conference, Sydney, Australia.

Castro, A., & Farmer, P. (2005). Understanding and addressing AIDS-related stigma: From anthropological theory to clinical practice in Haiti. *American Journal of Public Health, 95*(1), 53–59.

Chandra, P., Deepthivarma, S., & Manjula, V. (2003). Disclosure of HIV infection in south India: Patterns, reasons and reactions. *AIDS Care, 15*(2), 207–215.

Crewe, M., & Viljoen, F. (2005). *Testing times, routine HIV testing: A challenge to human rights.* Unpublished discussion paper, HIV Testing Discussion Group.

Csete, J., Shleifer, R., & Cohen, J. (2004). "Opt-out" testing for HIV in Africa: A caution. *The Lancet, 362*(9398), 1847–1849.

De Cock, K., Marum, E., & Mbori-Ngacha, D. (2002). Shadow on the continent: Public health and HIV/AIDS in Africa in the 21st century. *The Lancet, 360*(9326), 67–72.

De Cock, K., Marum, E., & Mbori-Ngacha, D. (2003). A serostatus-based approach to HIV/AIDS prevention and care in Africa. *The Lancet, 362*(9398), 1847–1849.

Global Business Coalition of HIV/AIDS. (2004). *The need to know: Accelerating access to testing.* Retrieved March 3, 2008, from http://www. businessfightsaids.org/site/pp.asp?c=gwKXJfNVJtF&b=1008763

Gruskin, S. (2004). Current issues and concerns in HIV testing: A health and human rights approach. *Canadian HIV/AIDS Policy and Law Review, 9*(3), 99–103.

Heywood, M. (2004). Human rights and HIV/AIDS in the context of 3 by 5: Time for new directions? *Canadian HIV/AIDS Policy and Law Review, 9*(2), 6–12.

Holbrooke, R. (2006, January 4). Sorry, but AIDS testing is critical. *Washington Post*, p. A17.

Holbrooke, R., & Furman, R. (2004, February 10). A global battle's missing weapon. *New York Times*, p. A25.

Kalichman, S., & Simbayi, L. (2004). Traditional beliefs about the cause of AIDS and AIDS-related stigma in South Africa. *AIDS Care, 16*(5), 572–580.

Kim, J. (2004, May 28). WHO's HIV/AIDS strategy under the spotlight. *In Focus: Online Bulletin of the WHO*, p. 1. Retrieved April 9, 2008, from http://www.who.int/bulletin/volumes/82/6/feature0604/en/

Kippax, S. (2006). A public health dilemma. *AIDS Care, 18*, 230–235.

Letamo, G. (2003). Prevalence of, and factors associated with, HIV/AIDS-related stigma and discriminatory attitudes in Botswana. *Journal of Health, Population and Nutrition, 21*(4), 347–357.

Maman, S., Mbwambo, J., Hogan, N., & Kilonzo, G. (2002). HIV-positive women report more lifetime partner violence: findings from a voluntary counselling and testing clinic in Dar es Salaam, Tanzania. *American Journal of Public Health, 92*(8), 1331–1337.

Mawar, N., Saha, S., Pandit, A., & Mahajan, U. (2005). The third phase of HIV pandemic: Social consequences of HIV/AIDS stigma & discrimination & future needs. *Indian Journal of Medical Research, 122*(6), 471–484.

McNaughton, M. (1992). HIV in women. *Early Human Development, 29*(103), 217–220.

Mill, J. (2003). Shrouded in secrecy: Breaking the news of HIV infection to Ghanaian women. *Journal of Transcultural Nursing, 14*(1), 6–16.

Muersing, K., & Sibind, F. (2000). HIV counselling—A luxury or necessity? *Health Policy and Planning, 15*(1), 17–23.

Mwamburi, D., Dladla, N., Qwana, E., & Lurie, M. (2005). Factors associated with wanting to know HIV results in South Africa. *AIDS Patient Care & STDs, 19*(8), 518–525.

Nems, M., Beaudoin, J., Conway, S., Kivumbi, G., Skjelmerud, A., & Vogel, U. (2006). *Evaluation of WHO's contribution to "3 by 5": Main report.* Geneva, Switzerland: WHO. Retrieved March 31, 2007, from http://www.who.int/hiv/topics/me/3by5evaluationreport.pdf

Nyblade, L., & Field-Nguer, M. (2001). *Women, communities and the prevention of mother-to-child transmission of HIV: Issues and findings from community research in Botswana and Zambia.* New York: International Centre for Research on Women. Retrieved March 31, 2007, from http://www.icrw.org/docs/mtct_2001_researchreport.pdf

Office of the Special Adviser for Africa (OSAA). (2004–2005). *Support for NEPAD; Period of report: August 2004–June 2005.* New York: United Nations Office of the Special Adviser for Africa. Retrieved March 7, 2008, from http://www.un.org/africa/osaa/2005%20UN%20System%20support%20for%20NEPAD/ECA.pdf

Office of the United States Global AIDS Coordinator. (2004). *The president's emergency plan for AIDS relief: US five year global HIV/AIDS strategy.* Washington, DC: Author.

Pignatelli S., Simpore, J., Pietra, V., Ouedraogo, L., Conombo, G., Saleri, N., et al. (2006). Factors predicting uptake of voluntary counselling and testing in a real-life setting in a mother-and-child center in Ouagadougou, Burkina Faso. *Tropical Medicine & International Health, 11*(3), 350–357.

Pizzi, M. (1992). Women HIV infection and AIDS: Tapestries of life, death and empowerment. *American Journal of Occupational Therapy, 46*(11), 1021–1027.

Rennie, S., & Behets, F. (2005). Desperately seeking targets: The ethics of routine HIV-testing in low-income countries. *Bulletin of the World Health Organization, 84*(1), 52–57.

Ross, E. (2004, July 10). U.N. experts call for routine HIV testing. *The Associated Press.* Retrieved March 31, 2007, from the UCLA Department of Epidemiology Web site: http://www.ph.ucla.edu/epi/seaids/routinetesting.html

Rubenstein, L. (2004, February 15). In the AIDS war, a call to arms [Letter to the editor]. *New York Times.* Retrieved March 2, 2008, from http://query.nytimes.com/gst/fullpage.html?res=9500E0D9163DF936 A25751C0A9629C8B63&partner=rssnyt&emc=rss

Seipone, K., Ntumy, R., Thuku, H., Mazhani, L., Creek, T., & Shaffer, N. (2004). Introduction of routine HIV testing in prenatal care—Botswana. *Morbidity and Mortality Weekly Report, 53*(46), 1083–1086.

Shane, V., & Kaplan, B. (1991). Double victims: Poor women and AIDS. *Women and Health, 17*(1), 21–37.

UNAIDS/WHO. (2004). *Policy statement on HIV testing: June 2004.* Geneva, Switzerland: UNAIDS/WHO. Retrieved March 31, 2007, from http://www.who.int/hiv/pub/vct/en/hivtestingpolicy04.pdf

United Nations. (2006). *Scaling up HIV prevention, treatment, care and support: Note by the Secretary-General.* New York: Author.

U.S. Department of State. (2004). *The president's emergency plan for AIDS relief: U.S. five-year global HIVAIDS strategy.* Washington, DC: United States Department of State.

Walton, D., Farmer, P., Lambert, W., Le' Andre, F., Koenig, S., & Mukherjee, J. (2004). Integrated HIV prevention and care strengthens primary health care: Lessons from rural Haiti. *Journal of Public Health Policy, 25*(2), 137–158.

World Health Organization (WHO). (2003). *Increasing access to HIV testing and counselling: report of a WHO consultation.* Geneva, Switzerland: Author. Retrieved March 31, 2007, from http://www.who.int/ hiv/pub/vct/en/IncreasingReportE.pdf

WHO TB/HIV Working Group. (2004). *Report of the 5th TB/HIV Core Group meeting.* Geneva, Switzerland: WHO. Retrieved March 31, 2007, from www.who.int/entity/tb/publications/tbhiv_addis_report/en

WHO/UNAIDS. (2003). *Treating 3 million by 2005: Making it happen.* Geneva, Switzerland: Author. Retrieved March 31, 2007, from http:// www.who.int/3by5/publications/documents/en/3by5StrategyMaking ItHappen.pdf

WHO/UNAIDS. (2004). *"3 by 5" progress report: December 2003 through June 2004.* Geneva, Switzerland: Author. Retrieved March 31, 2007, from http://www.who.int/3by5/en/Progressreport.pdf

WHO/UNAIDS. (2005). *"3 by 5" progress report: June 2005.* Geneva, Switzerland: Author. Retrieved March 31, 2007, from http://www. who.int/3by5/fullreportJune2005.pdf

WHO/UNAIDS. (2006). Progress on global access to HIV antiretoviral therapy: A report on "3 by 5" and beyond. Geneva, Switzerland: Author. Retrieved March 31, 2007, from http://www.who.int/hiv/ progreport2006_en.pdf

ENDNOTES

1. The Global Business Coalition of HIV/AIDS estimated in May 2004 that in order to meet the target of having 3 million people on ART by the end of 2005, "500,000 people will need to be tested each day" (p. 1).
2. Castro and Farmer (2005) argued convincingly that the notion of stigma tends to be individualized, and that the term "structural violence" is a more appropriate indication of the very real violence against HIV-positive people (pp. 54–55).

CHAPTER 9

"WE CRY FOR THE ORPHAN":

PICTURING AMERICAN GLOBAL CITIZENSHIP IN THE AIDS PANDEMIC

Meredith Raimondo

WHAT CONSCIENCE DEMANDS: AIDS AND THE AFRICAN ORPHAN

In a speech in advance of the 2005 G8 summit in Scotland, U.S. President George Bush spoke passionately about the United States' national concern for the impact of HIV in Africa:

> We seek progress in Africa and throughout the developing world because conscience demands it. Americans believe that human rights and the worth of human lives are not determined by race

or nationality, or diminished by distance. We believe that every
life matters and every person counts. And so we are moved when
thousands of young lives are ended every day by the treatable disease of malaria. We're moved when children watch their parents
slowly die of AIDS, leaving young boys and girls traumatized,
frightened and alone. Peoples of Africa are opposing these challenges with courage and determination and we will stand beside
them. (Bush, 2005)

At the heart of this drama of suffering and survival stands the "African
orphan," that tragic figure who evokes in an American audience a tide
of feeling powerful enough to close distance, create solidarity, and moti-
vate action.

Children, some of the epidemic's earliest and most visible "innocent victims,"[1] are not unfamiliar subjects in representations of AIDS.
In contemporary images of the AIDS pandemic in the U.S. media, the
suffering child invokes the magnitude, tragic effects, and dangerous possibilities emerging in the most affected regions of the world. It is this last
element—emerging danger—that suggests the inadequacy of innocence
to describe the discursive function of the child now.

In a 2002 story on AIDS in Africa entitled "A Continent of Orphans,"
the *Economist* warned that "A huge number of children without parental guidance is likely to spell trouble" (p. 41). What kind of trouble do
orphans cause for audiences constructed as remote—in terms of distance
and material conditions—from the lives of what human-rights advocates
term "children in difficult circumstances?" (UNESCO, 2002) This question provides an opportunity not just to reconsider the cultural work done
by images of the children in AIDS discourse, but also to examine the relationship between human rights, affect, and the militarization of health.
The last element may seem out of place in this sequence, evoking a violence at odds with feeling for the humanity of the suffering Other. However, the feelings evoked by the troubled and troublesome African orphan
construct a subject for whom these frameworks represent not oppositional, but rather enmeshed strategies for responding to global dangers.

Representations of children engage gender in complex ways. In the aforementioned examples, the child seems a subject free of gender, an aspect of adulthood not yet arrived. Indeed, the premature assumption of adult gender roles sometimes serves to indicate childhood defiled. What, then, constitutes a feminist engagement with the figure of the child and its effects in global AIDS discourse? In her influential *Bananas, Beaches, and Bases*, political scientist Cynthia Enloe (1990) proposed that a feminist approach to international relations might begin with the question, "where are the women?" (p. 7) While such an approach helpfully directs attention to the constitutive presences and absences in political discourse, it works most usefully as an opening into analysis, rather than as a methodology complete in itself. Images of children in AIDS discourse draw on gendered, raced, and classed logics, and construct the epidemic in highly gendered ways. While it is critical to observe the absence of women—indeed, of all adult caretakers—from the representation of bereft orphans, gender remains critical to the discourse of American caring. Feminist intervention into these representations requires an engagement, not just with the subjects of discourse, but also with the production of affect through the construction of subject positions. As cultural critic Lauren Berlant (1997) argued about "the Reaganite right," affect (she is specially concerned with sentiment) plays a central role in contemporary politics, "turn[ing] the nation into a privatized state of feeling" (p. 11). This essay considers one example in which the discourses of national feeling shapes engagement with global women's health.

I draw here in part on the work of AIDS cultural critics to draw attention to the politics of affect in media representations of the epidemic. Cindy Patton (1996), in a consideration of safe-sex education as "national pedagogy," argued that "the AIDS epidemic became a vehicle through which to renegotiate the meaning of being a good American" (pp. 7–10).[2] Literary critic Robert Corber (2003) explored a similar concern with affect, citizenship, and subject formation in his analysis of the 1993 film *Philadelphia*. He argued that the film's sentimental strategies for the recuperation of its central gay character serve as an example of a larger "psychification of national politics" (p. 114):

> Since the 1980s, sentimentality has operated in the mass-mediated public sphere as a technology of citizenship by mediating the deeply rooted racial, class, and gender conflicts that threaten to expose Reaganism's dismemberment of the national body. As a form of political pedagogy, it aims to instill in the national subject the 'right' way to feel about the groups whose disenfranchisement underlies her or his privilege. (p. 114)

Such arguments demonstrate the ways in which affect serves to reinforce inequalities in relationship to race, gender, sexuality, class, age, and other important axes of difference.

As U.S. media discourse about the African orphan suggests, such procedures of subject formation do not serve only to resolve conflicts internal to the nation. In the example of the Bush speech cited previously, feeling Americans also look beyond national borders, affirming their citizenship through their engagement with the world. Melani McAlister, in her 2001 study of U.S. representations of the Middle East, argued that "the politics of identity in the United States was intimately interwoven with the changing cultural logic of U.S. foreign policy," emerging in media "encounters" between American citizens and people and places they have never been (p. 42). Images of the AIDS pandemic, and especially Africa, have provided a crucial context for the articulation of American citizenship in a global context, inviting audiences to locate themselves on maps of risk and responsibility. Such representations engage the world in order to strengthen the boundaries of nation through the negotiation of spatial and temporal relations with variously constructed threatening Others.

In this essay, I consider the construction of affect in photojournalism from President Bush's widely publicized 2003 trip to Africa. The coupling of national interest and human rights in order to justify the amplification of U.S. global hegemony relies on an articulation of gendered subjectivities drawn from the heteronormative nuclear family. Such constructions do not function as mere metaphor, but serve to naturalize social, political, and economic inequalities as a necessary condition for the promotion of global security. I do not mean to suggest that this case exhausts the complex and even contradictory meanings that may inhere in the figure of the orphan as it circulates across diverse contexts, but rather to focus on one particular and highly visible set of images in order to illuminate the production of gendered, raced, and classed subjectivities that construct paternalism as a necessary and appropriate response to the global pandemic and leave progressive alternatives difficult to imagine. In this analysis, I want to express a critical skepticism about the apparent "progress" evident in the shift from a policy of disinterest to a policy of concern. Neocolonial sympathy for doomed women and their desperate children leaves intact the underlying structural inequalities that fuel the global AIDS pandemic and, in this case, promotes a militarization of international health discourse with potentially significant consequences for the very people such affective engagement is supposed to support. The adoption of human-rights rhetoric by the globally powerful in order to articulate violence as an ethical response to global dangers—seen also in the U.S. invasions of Afghanistan and Iraq—suggests that such frameworks may not, in the current moment, provide the political traction necessary to counter global hegemonies that render the pandemic as a natural rather than a political event.

"SOMETHING YOU'D NEVER SEE IN AMERICA": VISUAL INTIMACIES AND CITIZENSHIP

In July of 2003, U.S. President George Bush made a 5-day, five-nation tour of Senegal, South Africa, Botswana, Uganda, and Nigeria. The Bush administration used the carefully staged spectacle to highlight several policy initiatives, including economic development, the war on terror, and U.S. participation in the global response to AIDS. Reporters tended to describe the trip as an attempt to emphasize the administration's "compassionate conservativism" in the face of the largely negative international reception of U.S. unilateralism in Iraq.[3] Closer attention to the cultural work done by images of U.S. compassion suggests that it would be a mistake to see two contradictory forms of response to global crises at work in the defiant exercise of military might and a purported compassion towards people with AIDS. The Bush trip used the trope of the orphan to articulate the connections between these strategies for responding to perceived global dangers.

Acquired immune deficiency syndrome has become one of the critical features of the U.S. geographical imaginary in apocalyptic perceptions of "Africa" as a place both generative of, and emptied out by, epidemic disease (Johnson, 2002). Such constructions have done little to reveal any of the complex specificities of AIDS in the diverse contexts glossed as "Africa." Simon Watney (1994), for example, showed how popular narratives represented "'Africa' as an undifferentiated domain of rot, slime, filth, decay, disease, and naked 'animal' blackness" (p. 111). Similar logics shaped the obsessive interest in HIV's purported "African origin" in the 1980s, a construction that relied on a series of linked binary oppositions including black/white, primitive/civilized, animal/human, and diseased/sanitary.[4] These logics had significant material effects, shaping the direction of both research and policy in powerfully discriminatory ways.

The visibility of Africa in the 1980s was also a crucial component of U.S. media attempts to map what was routinely called the "spread of AIDS." Narratives mapping the global mobility of HIV invited U.S. readers and viewers to see their own futures in the apocryphal image of a devastated African continent.[5] In a work on cross-cultural representation, Elizabeth Hallam and Brian Street (2000) argued that "the ideological work of representation is often to translate social and cultural heterogeneity into homogenous unity and to emphasise boundaries which map zones of inclusion and exclusion" (Hallam & Street, 2000, pp. 6–7). "Africa," then, might be thought of less as a specific territory and more as the homogeneity produced through the circulation of images and narratives. Curtis Klein (1999) described the contours of that homogeneity by noting that "the overwhelming impression gained by studying American language about Africa seems to be that Africa is a primitive place, full of trouble and wild animals, and in need of our help" (p. 4).

Photographs also play an important role in such constructions, offering seemingly transparent evidence to the truth of such constructions.

Even a cursory examination of the three photo essays I discuss here—from CBS News, *Time*, and the U.S. Department of State—suggests that many of the tropes for representing AIDS in Africa in the 1980s remained in place in media coverage of Bush's 2003 trip, including primitivism, apocalypse, sexual perversity, and racialized violence.[6] However, instead of reading these images only as representations "of Africa," I want to treat them as opportunities to consider the production of U.S. citizenship. One indication of their interest in American identity is their almost obsessive preoccupation with President Bush, constructing opportunities for viewers to look at the president. These widely circulated images—or similar ones taken at carefully managed press conferences—construct a paternalistic U.S. citizenship in which caring justifies the exercise of global power. Global health inequalities provide an occasion not to consider feminist critiques of the bodily effects of transnational capitalism, but rather justify an intensification of global hegemony dependant on regressive hierarchies of gender, race, class, and nation.

The vast majority of the images of the tour focused on President Bush greeting crowds, meeting heads of state, touring sites, and seeing performances. "Africa" functioned as an uncanny mirror in which the only thing that could be seen clearly was Americanness. In this way, these photographs may be read in the context of a long history of travel narratives that imagine a foreign location as the site in which the meaning of nation can be most strongly felt.[7] Their invitation to viewers to travel with the president may seem, at first glance, to offer little more than a predictable colonial spectacle.

In a photograph taken in Uganda as part of a *Time* magazine photo essay (Kraft, 2003), a jet plane—an overdetermined marker of modernity—contrasts starkly with "traditionally" garbed figures in feathers and animal prints who have turned to watch it, "United States of America" framed between their headdresses (Kraft, image 11 of 12). Faceless, the figures appear as a colorful mass rather than as unique individuals. A bright red rope creates a literal border between them and Air Force One, leaving them crowded in the foreground while the plane, the subject of the image and the agent of this event, occupies the vast expanse of the tarmac. Yet still, the composition of the photograph troubles its own hierarchies, introducing a kind of uncertainty about the location of power. The figures in the foreground stand as tall as the plane, which is rendered small by distance and topped with a line of distant clouds that evoke both impending storm and explosion.[8] The red carpet is not a real barrier; it is incapable of holding back the crowd should it press forward. Both genial welcome and unanticipated violence are part of the colonial fantasy of encounter, and the construction of this image opens the possibility of either reading.

Of course, this reading depends on the legibility of Air Force One and the illegibility of the dress of those waiting for the plane. An audience familiar with the semiotics of the latter might find a very different meaning in the juxtaposition, perhaps even a conversation between modernities. The camera eye does not follow the Ugandans and their response to Bush, but tracks the president's travels to diverse nations and peoples whose particularities blur into an exotic backdrop for the familiar figure of American power. A number of images use the strategy of juxtaposing foreground and background to construct and reinforce binaries (Kraft, 2003, image 1 of 12).

In a photograph from the same event, dancing women—now in motion—tower over President Bush. The hand he holds up in greeting could also be a plea for the performers to maintain their distance. Such uncertainty simultaneously relies on and effaces the politics of race, gender, and class. The oppositional logic of these images posits Americanness against Africanness as a form of absolute alterity. Whiteness stands in contrast to blackness, and in this image, masculinity to femininity. Clothing serves as a cue for class relations. If the president's power suit stands for the expensively understated dress of Western gender-normative male elites, the colonial gaze of the camera situates the women's costumes in a premodern economy of handicraft that is rich in tradition but cash poor.[9] This construction of citizenship unmarks the president's whiteness, gender normativity, and economic privilege by subsuming them as signs of national identity. Distance in the photographs stands in for the distance of the viewer from the material location of these images, and opens the possibility that American power may be transformed into vulnerability—an ironic inversion in the context of health issues, where access to resources remains so unequally distributed.

Both photographs force the viewer to look through figures who are themselves gazing at the president. Thus, the viewer gazes at Others, but also gazes with them, troubling the boundary between subject and object. A similar dynamic is visible in an image from the tour of President Bush with President Mbeki in South Africa (Kraft, 2003, image 4 of 12).

A saluting figure in the foreground represents a potentially ambivalent site of identification for the viewer, as he looks towards the presidents and their wives, who are positioned in the background—which one does he salute? The Bushes have their hands on their hearts, moving this image squarely into the domain of American citizenship, but it is through the gaze of Africans that President Bush's Americanness is rendered visible.[10] The Bushes stand above the crowd, assembled to greet them in a position of power, but the building on whose steps they have emerged imposes a scale that renders them tiny. However, the image reveals little about the saluting person in the foreground, who is more a form than an individual. In the end, it is a photograph about the rituals of citizenship performed as a response to American power embodied in the president.

The ways in which these photographs invoke difference obscures rather than illuminates both historical and contemporary inequalities. This dynamic is clearly visible in media representations of the president's stop at Goree Island in Senegal, the first country visited on the trip.[11] This reckoning with the history of the transatlantic slave trade might have unsettled the binary opposition of Africa and America by foregrounding a long history of violent connections. Bush's speech managed to address and evade this history by lauding the heroism of enslaved peoples, celebrating "the stolen sons and daughters of Africa [that] helped to awaken the conscience of America. The very people traded into slavery helped to set America free"—a story about "my nation's journey toward justice" that avoided any acknowledgement of a national responsibility for historical and contemporary racial injustice by figuring the nation as enslaved rather than enslaving (Bush, 2003a).

Time's photo essay about the trip contained two images from this stop. In the first, Bush and Senegal's president, Abdoulaye Wadeand, stand in the doorway of what the caption identifies as "the slave house," gazing off into the distance. This first image, shot from below, positions the heads of state in opposition to a group of photographers, whose equipment almost seems like a barrier keeping Wadeand and Bush from advancing from the dark, confined doorway and into the sun (Kraft, 2003, image 2 of 12).

The second image is a cropped shot of the two men holding hands. It is a play in contrasts—Wadeand's white suit against Bush's dark suit is an ironic inversion that constructs race as a superficial difference rather than a historical and structural relation of power (Kraft, 2003, image 3 of 12). The clasped hands suggest intimacy, affection, equality, and, given the context of the stop to Goree Island, reconciliation.

This effacement of difference reveals how thoroughly such liberal humanist logics rely on race, gender, class, and sexual normativities. In the caption to this image, photographer Brooks Kraft (2003) noted that "Holding hands is a custom in Africa. It's not unusual for politicians to hold hands. But that's something you'd never see in America. You wouldn't see Bush and Bill Frist holding hands." This need to explain the clasped hands suggests an anxious disavowal of the possibility of something queer about the intimacy it represents. In light of the caption, the visibility of the wedding ring on Bush's left hand seems significant—does this suggest his immunity to the kinds of queer ways of seeing that Kraft's caption both recognizes and denies? The absence of the presidents' faces leaves the meaning of the clasped hands open-ended; there is no way for the viewer to know that the intimacy it promises is not erotic. Only "custom in Africa"—a promise that cultural identity is a site of absolute alterity—serves to recuperate its ambiguities. It is a binary that must be reasserted because it is not stable across these photographs—in the image of the salute discussed earlier (Kraft, 2003, image 4 of 12), for example, Africa seems to become America. The very instability of the binary's significance serves to foreground questions of nation, citizenship, and identity in these photographs.

In representing both Bush's performance as commander in chief and his experience of travel through "candid" reaction shots, the photo essays this chapter deals with simultaneously invoke diplomatic encounter and tourism. Each modality suggests a slightly differing form of identification with and meaning of the president. In his presidential modality, Bush is the embodiment of the nation itself—and as Dana Nelson and Tyler Curtain (2001) argued, to the extent that "the president stands in for United States democracy," there is a "collective longing for the power of the president" (p. 35). In this context, the figure of the president represents power that the individual citizen does not hold personally, but presumes to benefit from as a proper subject of the nation. In his tourist modality, Bush *is* the citizen, engaged in the familiar practice of collecting and disseminating visual souvenirs. The presumptive masculinity of the president as prototypical citizen is one way in which gender ideologies shape these images. The presence of Laura and Barbara Bush in some of the images further underscores this reading—these are images of the heteronormative family vacation. To the extent that these images evoke conventions of the family photo, they promote the viewer's identification. As Marianne Hirsch (1999) argued in her introduction to *The Familial Gaze*, "family pictures…are readily available for identification across the broadest and most radical divides" (p. xiii). What is shared in this case is both family and national identity—or perhaps more accurately, the identification with the family constructs an experience of national identity. As Nelson and Curtain (2001) pointed out, there is a widely shared "premise that the 'American family' is…the basic unit of American democracy" (p. 37).

Characterizing these images as vacation photos may seem to misrepresent the (public) genre of photojournalism as the (private) genre of family photography, but as Laura Wexler (2005) has persuasively argued, newspaper photography—a key site for the production of the nation—must be thought of in relation, rather than in contrast, to family photos: "The family portrait was a social practice which helped to a great extent to shape what was considered to be 'real' in the first place. It provided an excellent screen through which the news could be filtered" (pp. 101–102). Wendy Kozol's (2005) analysis of photojournalism in *Life* magazine provided a nuanced account of the ways in which representations of the family bridge rather than demarcate a rigid boundary between the political and the personal, demonstrating that "the public and private are interrelated rather that separate spheres" (p. 20). Foreign travel sometimes functions to demarcate a temporal and spatial distance from the domestic sphere of family, but the family vacation collapses these seemingly distinct times and spaces. In images of the Bush trip, tourism and diplomacy do not represent contradictory possibilities, but simultaneously present conventions that situate citizenship in an intimate realm, neither fully public nor fully private.

John Louis Lucaites and Robert Hariman (2001) argued that "the conventions of photojournalistic practice…situate the viewer in an emotional register that activates the tension between private and public life" (p. 41). While emotion is certainly central to the construction of subjects in the Bush photographs, the binary opposition of public and private fails to capture the ideological work of these images. Cultural critic Lauren Berlant (1997) has argued persuasively that citizenship in the United States no longer implies participation in the public sphere, but rather an affective domain that is "produced by personal acts and values, especially acts originating in or directed toward the family sphere" (p. 5). It is because these images of Bush evoke a familial context that they function so effectively as images of national identity. They also demonstrate that the family sphere operates at a range of scales. To engage in this form of citizenship is not always to withdraw into the private home or even domestic space defined by national borders. The citizenship these images produce does not stay at home, but acts globally.

Encounters with heads of state evoke domestic relations as a way of understanding the president's engagement with the people he meets; though official, they are also intimate. In one image, Ugandan President

Yoweri Museveni greets President Bush with Air Force One once again in the frame (U.S. Department of State, 2003, Uganda, 1st image). The positioning of three children between George and Laura Bush evokes not just diplomatic exchange but also the composition of family photographs, especially since Laura Bush is turned toward the children rather than toward the viewer. It is Museveni who appears to be the outsider in this image, entering the scene. Such representations construct for viewers an experience of paternalism in which the intimacy of family forms serves as a model for understanding the relationship between nations, installing gender hierarchies as an natural feature of political engagement.

"SOME WITH THE HIV VIRUS": MOTHERS, ORPHANS, AND AIDS

In remarks made during his stop in Botswana that were widely reported by U.S. media,[12] Bush stated, "the American people care deeply about the pandemic that sweeps across this continent, the pandemic of HIV/AIDS…We cry for the orphan…we cry for the mom who is alone" (Bush, 2003b). While women and children have long embodied the feminized, vulnerable "victims" of AIDS, photographs from the tour represent a shift from images of the wasted, sick, visibly ill bodies in distress that have traditionally buttressed a paternalistic U.S. view of AIDS in Africa. Instead, the images situate President Bush in and among women and children, often touching them directly in a relationship of caring proximity rather than a disembodied distant gaze.

In a photograph of the Bushes clasping raised hands with singers and employees of TASO, an AIDS service organization in Uganda, the convergence of horizontal lines on the walls and ceiling directs the viewer's gaze toward the president, constructing him as the opposite—and the mirror—of the viewer's imagined position in the circle, hands raised with imagined African neighbors (Sterner, 2003).

Images of the president with children focused centrally on the production of an affective response to orphans. In Uganda, as the *New York Times* reported,

Mr. Bush heard a moving rendition of "America the Beautiful" by a choir of children who had lost one or both parents to AIDS or to war. They finished the song with broad smiles on their faces and their arms stretched toward heaven. (Stevenson, 2003)

In an image of the performance by the choir discussed in the aforementioned quotation (U.S. Department of State, 2003, Uganda, 3rd image), Bush does not look at the camera, seemingly captured in a candid moment of surprise and pleasure. This framing returns the focus to Bush, emphasizing his reaction to the children rather than to the event itself.

In another photograph of the same event (Kraft, 2003, image 12 of 12), the children are slightly out of focus, providing an almost dreamlike (perhaps even heavenly?) background for Bush, who points at the camera as if to draw the viewer into the scene and demand that they, like he, take notice. It is not their appeal but the president's that the viewer must engage.

The image of heaven/salvation suggests the role of evangelical missionaries in the circulation of images of African children in the United States.[13] Christian charitable organizations rely extensively on visual imagery to solicit funds for sponsorship programs, which promise a relationship with an individual needy child in return for donations. Photographs play a critical role in such campaigns, both to personalize need and to reward giving, seeming to provide a medium that transcends distance, literacy, and language barriers. Such appeals rely heavily on the power of images to incite such strong feeling, that action—in this case, donation—is the only tolerable response.

Images of adult women with AIDS have also served an important role in constructing Africa as a continent of orphans for which Americans will assume responsibility. Photographs from a meeting of the Bushes with women with AIDS in Nigeria seem to flirt with the discourse of transracial adoption, in which the economically privileged, white, heterosexual couple rescues needy children from a fate their mothers cannot escape. As Sandra Patton (2000) argued, transracial adoption—once a suspect practice related to challenges around cultural identities—emerged in policy discourse in the 1990s as a potential solution to racialized poverty.

Social rhetoric pathologized African American families (and especially African American mothers) for "endangering the whole of society by failing to socialize 'productive' citizens" (Patton, p. 169). Patton pointed to a barely subsumed religious rhetoric in adoption discourse:

> Transracial adoption provides the quality of salvation and redemption to this story. Not only does it representationally provide for the "salvation" of inner-city Black children, but it also allows for the "redemption" of Whites from the "burdens" of racism and guilt by affirming as "color-blind" and antiracist those politicians and advocates who favor transracial placements and Whites who adopt Black children. (p. 182)

In the transnational context of the global AIDS pandemic, "illegitimacy"—as a marker of antinational, racialized sexualities and deviant family forms—does not play the same role that Patton argued it does in the United States. Instead, AIDS serves as the mark of racialized sexual danger whose social effects can be ameliorated through the production of nuclear families characterized by sexual fidelity.

Images of the president with women and their children also emphasize caring, connection, and bodily proximity. In a U.S. Department of State (2003, Nigeria, 6th image) Web site photo of the Bushes meeting women in Nigeria, neither the Bushes nor the unnamed women gaze directly into the camera, though the positioning of the Bushes slightly behind the women, combined with their height and upward gaze, creates a visual hierarchy. The child's head is turned towards Laura Bush, constructing a connection between the foreground and background that draws the viewer's gaze towards the First Lady.

In another image from the same meeting in Nigeria (U.S. Department of State, 2003, Nigeria, 5th image), Bush clasps hands with one of the mothers as her child and other women gaze at him smiling from the background. The clasped hands—both a symbol of greeting and a symbol of agreement—are the focus of the image, caught in the gaze of the peering child.

A photo (U.S. Department of State, 2003, Uganda, 2nd image) of Bush meeting clients of a Ugandan AIDS organization shows a similar pattern—as he bends over to speak to a woman in a blue shirt, the child in front of her ends up framed in his arms. First Lady Laura Bush also plays an important role in these images of the compassionate American, suggesting that its affective dimensions are complexly gendered.

The overdetermined maternalism in photographs of reading aloud (U.S. Department of State, 2003, Uganda, 5th image) and doll making (U.S. Department of State, Botswana, 5th image) fills the gap left by dying mothers. At their most pernicious, such missionary images can be read to suggest that the sundering of families might be a form of social good, liberating children from the diseased premodernity of their mothers through the benevolent neocolonial caring of U.S. global hegemony.

However, orphans are not always stable signifiers of innocence—they also, as the *Economist* warned, "spell trouble," representing the possibility of chaos ("Forty Million Orphans," 2002, p. 41).

In an photograph that appeared on the U.S. Department of State Web site, (U.S. Department of State, 2003, Uganda, 4th image), for example, Laura Bush sits among stiffly posed children who stand close around her, forcing her to lean to the side to be visible to the camera. The image's composition is familiar, almost banal, suggesting the grade-school class photo. Surrounded by a crowd of children, the seated Bush must lean informally to the side to be seen, smiling broadly as she embodies a comfort with proximity. However, as I have suggested, apparently happy crowds can have multiple meanings in the racist colonial imaginary. In this case, the caption of the image seems to excavate possibilities not visually available. Reading simply, "Ugandan school children, some with the HIV virus" (U.S. Department of State), this textual elaboration invites the viewer to consider which of the somber children are living with HIV without visually providing any clues to their identity. The resulting uncertainty, which combines long-standing tropes about the difficulty of identifying dangerous "AIDS carriers" and the representation of Africa as the unknowable "dark continent," suggests the locus where the discourse of parental compassion meets the discourse of threatened security. Is Laura Bush the protector here, or is she the one in need of protection? Unlike Bush, the children do not smile, their stiff faces providing no clue to their reaction to her. The invisibility of HIV serves as a metaphor for the unknown dangers even children can harbor.

The casual touches offered by the president and first lady suggest that the danger of AIDS to Americans is not to be found in bodily proximity to Africans. Instead, the possibility of a land of orphans suggests the potential for a dangerous future, the question of what might happen in the moment just beyond the one captured in the photograph.

Consider an image of President Bush meeting children during his arrival in Botswana (U.S. Department of State, 2003, Botswana, 1st image). Children hold flags from both countries, but in both cases, Botswana's flag is more visible, covering the U.S. flag and raised over it. The smiles and the sense of action created by the tangled, reaching hands suggest high spirits, but the crowding might also signify the formation of a mob threatening to swallow Bush as the reporters, visible in the corner with a camera, look on. In another image from the Ugandan performance, the children appear on the verge of engulfing the president. The animal prints of their clothes, with no cultural context to suggest their value and meaning, encode a kind of potential menace into the image, coupling affection with appetite (CBS News, 2003, image 18 of 12).

Of course, it is entirely possible to look at these images and see the joyful event that is clearly their intended meaning. Nonetheless, all three images (CBS News, 2003, image 18 of 12; U.S. Department of State, 2003, Botswana, 1st image, Uganda, 4th image) feature crowds of children that can be read in more ominous ways. The images foreclose neither reading, nor even a simultaneous experience of multiple possibilities in the same scene.

For viewers who encountered these images in the context of print-media coverage of the trip, the tension between the transparency of good will and unseen dangers may have been further heightened by the widespread discussion of Africa as a potential site for terrorist activity. Perhaps in recognition of the intensification of armed conflict in Liberia during Bush's tour, journalists used Africa as a key site for evaluating the risk of what policy analysts describe as "failed states."[14] In this coverage, orphans were not only the victims of AIDS but also its potential monsters. What might they become, bereft of both individual families and the disciplinary structure of statehood?[15] An *Atlanta Journal-Constitution* editorial mused,

> In an interconnected world of AIDS, terrorism, and other threats, a policy of malign indifference is no longer possible. If the West does not share its peace and prosperity with Africa, Africa will share its despair and anguish with the West. ("Involvement With Africa," 2003, p. A10)

"Failed states," newspapers noted again and again, serve as "reservoirs" and "breeding grounds" for terrorism—precisely the same language newspapers used to describe Africa as the generative source of AIDS.[16]

Conscious of such dangers, the paternalistic global citizenship constructed in these representations of Bush's African tour did not merely invite compassion, but also the exercise of discipline.[17] In the coverage of Bush's trip, compassion and military action represent related strategies for preventing dangerous vectors from escaping their breeding grounds to threaten the vulnerable national citizen, another example of the ways in which, as Amy Kaplan (2003) has argued, domestic space must be protected from beyond the nation's borders. Because the images in question invite the viewer simultaneously to identify with the caring U.S. parent and with the child-like African, the logic of compassionate discipline takes on a self-reinforcing circularity. As the vulnerable child, we find comfort in the empowered but caring parent; as the compassionate parent, we know our discipline to be rooted in the compassion we feel towards the child. Such tropes are incoherent without gendered hierarchies that simultaneously naturalize both inequality and particular forms of kinship. When international relations are contained in such familial metaphors, war is not visible as war, because an orphaned world desperately needs the compassionate hand of paternal discipline. For the militarized American citizen such circumstances demand, the violent exercise of power represents a sensitive, affective response to variously situated vulnerabilities.

It goes without saying that this discourse of American citizenship depends centrally on, and serves to reinforce, the very constructions of difference it purports to overcome, further reinforcing hierarchies of race, class, gender, sexuality, and national identity in the guise of a transcendent humanism that reaches out to intervene in Africa, even as the populations most affected by AIDS within the United States find themselves increasingly unable to access medical care, social services, or basic material needs.[18] The familial dynamics of U.S. paternalistic global citizenship naturalize these historical inequalities as not only inevitable, but indeed, necessary to the production of global order and domestic security.

"A DEADLIER GLOBAL THREAT": HUMAN RIGHTS AND THE "WAR ON AIDS"

> In Africa, promise and opportunity sit side by side with disease, war, and desperate poverty. This threatens both a core value of the United States—preserving human dignity—and our strategic priority—combating global terror. American interests and American principles, therefore, lead in the same direction: we will work with others for an African continent that lives in liberty, peace, and growing prosperity.
>
> —White House Africa Policy (2006)

In the months following September 11, 2001, editorials in the activist, social-service, community-based, and even mass media worried about the impact of the new "war on terror" on AIDS prevention and treatment. With public and private funding priorities in a state of unanticipated upheaval and redirection, the outlook seemed bleak, especially as the much trumpeted "war chest" of the Global Fund to Fight AIDS, Tuberculosis, and Malaria failed to fill. Writing in *The Nation*, Africa Action executive director Salih Booker (2002) presented the situation bluntly:

> Whether measured by numbers killed or nations wounded, by economies upended or families crushed, the AIDS pandemic is

a deadlier global threat than that posed by terrorist groups. But almost no one draws the logical conclusion: The war on AIDS is more important than the war on terrorism. Those on the frontlines of this war—people living with AIDS, medical professionals and community activists, family and friends—are fighting back with the meager resources they have. Report after report documents what needs to be done. The price tag is modest compared with the sums quickly appropriated in response to September 11. Yet only a trickle of resources is reaching the AIDS battle fronts...Years from now people will ask about AIDS, as with the Holocaust or the Rwandan genocide, "How could they have known—and failed to act?" (n.p.)

Booker's militarized rhetoric is striking, but his final question suggests the context for this stirring call to arms. The reference to both the Holocaust and the Rwandan genocide suggests his investment in a human-rights frame that constructs failure to act as a profound moral wrongdoing. Offered as a critique of U.S. policy, both of these historical cases underscore nonaction as a form of culpability that violated the right to life of the victims of genocide.

Six years later, the relationship between the war on terror and the U.S. response to AIDS remains unclear—including the extent to which they ought be thought of as projects in opposition. The same administration responsible for the invasions of Afghanistan and Iraq and the incarcerations at Guantanamo Bay and elsewhere has also paid consistent, perhaps unprecedented, attention to the global AIDS pandemic. The president's Emergency Plan for AIDS Relief, announced in the 2003 State of the Union address, called for new levels of U.S. participation in the global response to HIV/AIDS. For much of the first part of the U.S. epidemic, AIDS activists defined official indifference, indicated by the inaction of federal, state, and local governments, as one of their central challenges. Now, it is official involvement that represents an important source of concern. The direction of funding to abstinence-only prevention programs, the retention of federal control of appropriations in lieu of donations to more socially progressive U.N.-funded programs, and the pressures on sexually explicit research and programming (especially directed at gay men and sex workers) are all examples of the vast gap between federal policy and the needs of community activists and organizers.

What has clearly changed is the symbolic politics of presidential concern. The visibility of AIDS has transformed dramatically since the 1980s, when activists pointed to President Reagan's silence as evidence of broader disregard for the AIDS crisis. President Bush speaks often and passionately about AIDS., and increasingly, he uses the language of human rights to characterize the problem of AIDS, and to suggest the necessity of a U.S. response. The adoption of human-rights frames by global elites demonstrates, in part, the success of transnational AIDS activists in changing the terms of the debate. In the 1990s, human-rights framings of HIV provided an important strategy for progressive activists, researchers, and policy makers to articulate the relationship between HIV infection and social and structural inequality (Farmer, 2003; Gostin & Lazzarini, 1997; Mann & Tarantola, 1992, 1996; Petchesky, 2003). This lens challenged narrow, biomedical framings of AIDS, emphasizing the importance of understanding the lethal consequences of colonial legacies, the brutalities of contemporary economic globalization, and the everyday abrogation of the right to life by the global status quo. Its normative stance offered a tool to challenge the powerful to take responsibility for the conditions that transformed the pandemic into a political crisis, and demanded action to ameliorate the conditions that left too many vulnerable to preventable infection and early death.

In his influential remapping of the concept of power, Michel Foucault (1990) proposed that "Power is not an institution, and not a structure; neither is it a certain strength we are endowed with; it is the name that one attributes to a complex strategical situation in a particular society" (p. 93). Foucault's formulation characterizes power not as a static object, but rather as an aggregative "effect," simultaneously forceful and unstable. It also suggests the necessity of thinking of resistance as tactical, able to respond to the often unpredictable and sometimes dizzying shifts that characterize relations of power. As Cindy Patton (1996) observed in her analysis of safe sex education, "if the state is more diffuse than activists of the 1980s imagined, then the efforts and effects of their projects must have been less clearly oppositional than neo-Marxian analysis suggested, less predictable than neopositive sociologists hoped" (p. 9).

Though human rights have been a vitally important tool in particular contexts—and particularly useful for reframing gender inequalities as social and structural rather than simply intimate and individual—a human-rights frame does not offer a stable location from which to critique global hegemony. At this moment, it may not serve to think about human rights and militarism as distinct and oppositional discourses, different forms of political globalization competing to shape the development of policy priorities and the distribution of resources. Ongoing U.S. military intervention in Afghanistan and Iraq illustrates the ways in which human rights—and especially women's human rights—are increasingly invoked to support global hegemonies, particularly that of U.S. militaristic/capitalist dominance. In the context of the AIDS pandemic, human-rights frames are also being appropriated for very different ends than their progressive advocates would hope. To ask whether U.S. policy attends more to the war on terror or to the response to AIDS is to miss the ways these projects have converged.

A cynical reading, attentive to the gap between lofty words and destructive policies, might simply dismiss Bush's human-rights rhetoric as predictable hypocrisy, a use of noble-sounding words to justify oppressive acts. It would be easy—perhaps even tempting—to dismiss his mawkish invocation of suffering children and their dying mothers as a cynical attempt to construct a neocolonialist human drama, in order to obscure the underlying structural violence of global poverty and its relationship to the uneven distribution of infectious disease. Such a critique defines the central problem as one of dishonesty—the problem is not in the frame but in its disingenuous use. Given the easy convergence of the human-rights commitment to the right to life with the evangelical culture of life so central to the policy discourse of the Bush Administration, accusations of insincerity seem inadequate for this political moment. It may be that when the president reports feeling moved, he means what he says, and it may be that some of his listeners are moved with him, in a response quite at odds with the notion of compassion fatigue.[19] Human-rights frames engage directly in the process of subject formation through practices of identification and feeling. When coupled with discourses of citizenship that emphasize vulnerability, powerlessness, and loss, they may serve to reinforce the very global hegemonies that continue to produce and distribute different forms of illness, danger, and untimely death. Feminist considerations of the construction of gendered subjectivities suggest the urgent need to develop a critical stance that will serve to challenge oppressive power relations, not in a context of callous disinterest, but in one of sincere feelings for suffering Others. As these racialized, gendered, and nationalized images of AIDS suggest, these discourses may play an important role in shaping what it is possible to do—or even what it is possible to think—about women's health.

REFERENCES

Berlant, L. (1997). *The Queen of America goes to Washington City: Essays on sex and citizenship.* Durham, NC: Duke University Press.

Blunt, A. (1994), *Travel, gender, and imperialism: Mary Kingsley and West Africa.* New York: The Guilford Press.

Booker, S. (2002, January 7). AIDS: Another world war. *The Nation.* Retrieved June 2, 2005, from http://www.thenation.com

Bush, G. (2003a, July 8). *President speaks at Goree Island in Senegal. Speech at Goree Island, Senegal.* Retrieved October 10, 2005, from http://www.whitehouse.gov/news/releases/2003/07/20030708-1.html

Bush, G. (2003b, July 10). *President discusses AIDS initiative and Iraq in Botswana. Remarks and photo opportunity with Botswanan President Mogae in Gaberone, Botswana.* Retrieved October 10, 2005, from http://www.whitehouse.gov/news/releases/2003/07/20030710-3.html

Bush, G. (2005, June 30). *President discusses G-8 summit and progress in Africa. Speech to the Hudson Institute, at the Freer Gallery, Washington, DC.* Retrieved October 10, 2005, from http://www.whitehouse.gov/news/releases/2005/06/20050630.html

Cardelle, R., Drainoni, M., Harris, V., Mancusi, M., Mayo, J., Schluter, D., et al. (2004). Service-system gaps for people with HIV/AIDS and additional health challenges. *AIDS & Public Policy Journal, 19*(3/4), 110–112.

CBS News. (2003). *Trip to Africa* [Photo essay]. Retrieved October 12, 2005, from http://www.cbsnews.com/elements/2003/07/10/in_depth_photos/photoessay562607.html

Chirimuuta, R., & Chirimuuta, R. (1989), *AIDS, Africa and racism.* London: Free Association Books.

Corber, R. (2003). Nationalizing the gay body: AIDS and sentimental pedagogy. *American Literary History, 15,* 107–133.

Deans, B. (2003, July 6). Conflict, critics shadow Bush. *Atlanta Journal-Constitution,* p. A4.

Donnelly, J. (2003, July 11). Bush promises US help in Africa's AIDS battle. *Boston Globe*, p. A8.

Duncan J., & Gregory, D. (Eds.). (2000). *Writes of passage: Reading travel writing*. New York: Routledge.

Edelman, L. (2004). *No future: Queer theory and the death drive*. Durham, NC: Duke University Press.

Engle, J. (2003, July 11). Bush visit shuts down Senegal. *The Nation*. Retrieved March 19, 2008, from http://www.thenation.com/doc/20030804/engle

Enloe, C. (1990). *Bananas, beaches, and bases: Making feminist sense of international politics*. Berkeley, CA: University of California Press.

Farmer, P. (2003). *Pathologies of power: Health, human rights, and the new war on the poor*. Berkeley, CA: University of California Press.

Forty million orphans. (2002, November 30). *The Economist*, p. 41. Retrieved October 12, 2005, from the Academic Search Premier Database.

Foucault, M. (1990). *The history of sexuality: An introduction* (Vol. 1). New York: Vintage Books.

Gikandi, S. (1996). *Maps of Englishness: Writing identity in the culture of colonialism*. New York: Columbia University Press.

Gostin, L., & Lazzarini, Z. (1997). *Human rights and public health in the AIDS pandemic*. New York: Oxford University Press.

Grover, J. (1988). AIDS: Keywords. In D. Crimp (Ed.), *AIDS: Cultural analysis, cultural criticism* (pp. 29–30). Cambridge, MA: The MIT Press.

Hagos, A. (2000). *Hardened images: The Western media and the marginalization of Africa*. Trenton, NJ: Africa World Press.

Hallam, E., & Street, B. (2000). Introduction. In E. Hallam & B. Street (Eds.), *Cultural encounters: Representing "Otherness"* (pp. 1–10). New York: Routledge.

Hammonds, E. (2001). Missing persons: African American women, AIDS, and the history of disease. In K. Hogan (Ed.), *Women take care: Gender, race, and the culture of AIDS* (pp. 7–23). Ithaca, NY: Cornell University Press.

Haraway, D. (1994). Teddy bear patriarchy: Taxidermy in the garden of Eden, New York City, 1908–36. In A. Kaplan & D. Pease (Eds.), *Cultures of United States imperialism* (pp. 237–291). Durham, NC: Duke University Press.

Heslin, K. et al. (2005). Racial and ethnic disparities in access to physicians with HIV-related expertise. *Journal of General Internal Medicine, 20*(3), 283–289.

Hickey, D., & Wylie, K. (1993). *An enchanting darkness: The American vision of Africa in the twentieth century.* East Lansing, MI: Michigan State University Press.

Hirsch, M. (1999). Introduction: Familial looking. In M. Hirsch (Ed.), *The familial gaze* (pp. xi–xxv). Hanover, NH: Dartmouth College.

Hogan, K. (2001). *Women take care: Gender, race, and the culture of AIDS.* Ithaca, NY: Cornell University Press.

Involvement with Africa is in America's best interest [Editorial]. (2003, July 8). *Atlanta Journal-Constitution,* p. A10.

Johnson, K. (2002). AIDS as U.S. national security threat: Media effects and geographical imaginations. *Feminist Media Studies, 2*(1), 81–96.

Kaplan, A. (2003). Homeland insecurities: Reflections on language and space. *Radical History Review, 85*(1), 82–93.

Kemper, B. (2003, July 11) Bush reaffirms AIDS pledge in Botswana. *Chicago Tribune,* pp. A1–A3.

Klein, C. (1999). *Mistaking Africa: Curiosities and inventions of the American mind.* Boulder, CO: Westview Press.

Kozol, W. (2003, October 17). *Anxiety and comfort under the mushroom cloud: Masculinity, militarism, and national belonging.* Paper presented to the American Studies Association Annual Meeting, Hartford, CT.

Kozol, W. (2005). "The kind of people who make good Americans": Nationalism and *Life's* family ideal. In A. Cameron (Ed.), *Looking for America: The visual production of nation and people* (pp. 173–211). Malden, MA: Blackwell Publishing.

Kraft, B. (2003, July 18). Following President Bush. *Time.* Retrieved October 10, 2005, from http://www.time.com/time/photoessays/bushafrica/

Krasner, S., & Pascual, C. (2005). Addressing state failure. *Foreign Affairs, 84*(4), 153–163.

Lucaites, J., & Hairman, R. (2001). Visual rhetoric, photojournalism, and democratic public culture. *Rhetoric Review, 20*(1/2), 37–42.

Mann, J., & Tarantola, D. (1992). *AIDS in the World.* Cambridge, MA: Harvard University Press.

Mann, J., & Tarantola, D. (1996). *AIDS in the World II.* New York: Oxford University Press.

McAlister, M. (2001). *Epic encounters: Culture, media, and U.S. interests in the Middle East, 1945–2000.* Berkeley. CA: California University Press.

Melvin, D. (2003, July 6). Bush carries AIDS plan to Africa. *Atlanta Journal-Constitution*, p. 5A.

Moeller, S. (1999). *Compassion fatigue: How the media sell disease, famine, war and death.* New York: Routledge.

Morales, L. S., Cunningham, W. E., Galvan, F. H., Andersen, R. M., Nakazono, T. T., & Shapiro, M. F. (2004). Sociodemographic differences in access to care among Hispanic patients who are HIV infected in the United States. *American Journal of Public Health, 94*(7), 1119–1121.

Nelson, D., & Curtain, T. (2001). The symbolics of presidentialism. In L. Berlant & L. Duggan (Eds.), *Our Monica, ourselves: The Clinton affair and the national interest* (pp. 34–52). New York: New York University Press.

Patton, C. (1990). *Inventing AIDS.* New York: Routledge.

Patton, C. (1996). *Fatal advice: How safe-sex education went wrong.* Durham, NC: Duke University Press.

Patton, S. (2000). *Birth marks: Transracial adoption in contemporary America.* New York: New York University Press.

Petchesky, R. (2003). *Global prescriptions: Gendering health and human rights.* New York: Zed Books.

Raimondo, M. (1999). *The next wave: Media maps of the "spread of AIDS."* Unpublished doctoral dissertation, Emory University, Atlanta, GA.

Raimondo, M. (1999). Corralling the virus: Migratory sexualities and the spread of AIDS. *Environment and Planning D: Society and Space, 21*(4), 389–407.

Reuters. (2003, August 31). *Liberia's child soldiers struggle to rebuild lives.* Retrieved September 14, 2006, from CNN Web site: http://edition.cnn.com/2003/WORLD/africa/08/31/liberia.child.soldiers.reut/

Roth, B. (2003, July 11). Message delivered. *Houston Chronicle,* p. A21.

Siegel, K. (Ed.) (2002). *Issues in travel writing: Empire, spectacle, and displacement.* New York: Peter Lang.

Sterner, S. (2003, July 11). President George W. Bush, Mrs. Laura Bush, and to the president's right, Ugandan President Yoweri Museveni and Mrs. Museveni sing along with a choir and staff members of The AIDS Support Organization (TASO) Centre in Entebbe, Uganda. *White House News and Policies.* Retrieved October 10, 2005, from http://www.whitehouse.gov/news/releases/2003/07/images/20030712_uganda1-515h.html

Stevenson, R. (2003, July 12). Bush has praise for Uganda in its fight against AIDS. *New York Times,* p. A4.

Sweet, L. (2003, July 8). Africa suddenly front-and-center. *Chicago Sun-Times,* p. A6.

Thomma, S. (2003). Bush vows help on AIDS. *Milwaukee Journal Sentinel,* p. A3.

Treichler, R. (1999). *How to have theory in an epidemic.* Durham, NC: Duke University Press.

UNESCO. (2002). *Children in difficult circumstances: Strengthening partnerships to combat HIV/AIDS and discrimination.* Paris: Author, Programme of Education for Children in Difficult Circumstances. Retrieved March 19, 2008, from http://unesdoc.unesco.org/images/0012/001293/129349e.pdf

U.S. Department of State. (2003). *President Bush's trip to Africa, July 7–12, 2003.* Retrieved October 10, 2005, from http://usinfo.state.gov/regional/af/potus2003/gallery/photogallery.htm

Walsh, K. (2003, July 21). Bush on the wild side. *U.S. News and World Report*, p. 10.

Watney, S. (1994). *Practices of freedom: Selected writings on HIV/AIDS.* Durham, NC: Duke University Press.

Wexler, L. (2005). Techniques of the imaginary nation: Engendering family photography. In A. Cameron (Ed.), *Looking for America: The Visual Production of Nation and People* (pp. 94–117). Malden, MA: Blackwell Publishing.

White House Africa Policy. (2006). Retrieved May 25, 2005, from http://www.whitehouse.gov/infocus/africa/

ENDNOTES

1. Jan Zita Grover (1988) discussed the child as innocent victim in "AIDS: Keywords," in *AIDS: Cultural Analysis, Cultural Criticism*. Cindy Patton (1996) considers the trope of innocence in relation to the child extensively in *Fatal Advice: How Safe-Sex Education Went Wrong* (see especially chapters 2 and 3). Like Patton, Katie Hogan (2001) considered the racialization of this trope in *Women Take Care: Gender, Race, and the Culture of AIDS* (see especially chapter 3). Hogan's work is indebted to the groundbreaking analysis of African American women with HIV and discourses of child endangerment by Evelynn Hammonds (2001) in "Missing persons: African American women, AIDS, and the history of disease." Clearly, representations of children as iconic figures have far-reaching effects in American political culture. In *The Queen of America Goes to Washington City: Essays on Sex and Citizenship*, Lauren Berlant (1997) argued that

   > when social-welfare policies can be justified only for the sake of 'the children,' we know that the political imagination's displacement away from adults to the horizon of 'our children' or the 'unborn' signifies a widespread incapacity to conceive, with the overabundance of information we already have, a positive sense of the present or the future of the adult American. (p. 143)

   In *No Future: Queer Theory and the Death Drive*, Lee Edelman (2004) proposed that "the Child, that is, marks the fetishistic fixation of heteronormativity: an erotically charged investment in the rigid sameness of identity that is central to the compulsory narrative of reproductive futurism" (p. 21). While these arguments forcefully reveal the ways in which the figure of the child functions to police queerness and promote heteronormativity, the orphan—who is, after all, not the "own" child but the Other's child—may suggest the need to integrate these kinds of queer critiques more thoroughly with postcolonial and antiracist analysis.

2. Patton (1996) demonstrated the evolution of the unmarked, normatively white, middle-class, heterosexual "general public," fearful of contamination by dangerous deviants, into the "compassionate citizen," whose feelings for the person with AIDS serve as evidence of his or her distance from the risk of infection (see pp. 20, 21).

3. The *Atlanta Journal-Constitution* reported that Bush's purpose included "softening his warrior image at home and abroad" (Deans, 2003, p. A4).

4. For further discussion of representations of "African AIDS," see Paula Treichler's (1999) *How to Have Theory in an Epidemic*, and Cindy Patton's (1990) *Inventing AIDS*.

5. I have discussed media representations of the "spread of AIDS" in more detail elsewhere. See M. Raimondo's (2003) "Corralling the Virus: Migratory Sexualities and the Spread of AIDS."

6. Lest the association of Africa with animals seem an oversimplification, it seems worth noting that President Bush managed to find time for the requisite visit to a nature reserve on his brief trip. In the carefully stage-managed spectacle of the tour, the stop at the Mokolodi Nature Reserve in Botswana provided one of the few breaks in the script. In an incident widely reported in the international press and joked about on late-night television in the United States, one of the elephants brought out for display mounted another. Most coverage emphasized the President's enjoyment of the moment, including a bawdy comment directed at his wife. In a photograph of the event, the Bushes and a guide are captured in an open pickup, the elephants to the right of the frame. The others have their backs to the camera, but Bush looks over his shoulder to meet the viewer's gaze with a knowing smirk—a subjectivity constructed through this scene of colonial encounter, juxtaposing the unrestrained erotics of nature with domesticated white femininity (see K. Walsh, 2003). The production of normative heterosexuality and masculinity through this eruption of undomesticated sexuality might be taken as a 21st-century version of the politics of national identity production through (presidential) encounters with the African elephant. See Donna Haraway's (1994) critique, "Teddy Bear Patriarchy: Taxidermy in the Garden of Eden, New York City, 1908–36."

7. A critical tradition has developed that examines representations of Africa for their accuracy or inaccuracy. See, for example, Richard Chirimuuta and Rosalind Chirimuuta (1989), *AIDS, Africa and Racism* (Free Association Books); Asgede Hagos (2000), *Hardened Images: The Western Media and the Marginalization of Africa*; or Dennis Hickey and Kenneth Wylie (1993), *An Enchanting Darkness: The American Vision of Africa in the Twentieth Century*. While this work illustrates one important strategy for the critique of such problematic ideologies, I am more influenced here by travel theorists, who take the inaccuracy, colonialism, racism, and/or romanticism that so often structure Western accounts of journeys to cultural

and geographic Others not as their conclusion, but as an opening for a consideration of the ideologies of identity such representations produce. For example, Simon Gikandi noted in his 1996 *Maps of Englishness: Writing Identity in the Culture of Colonialism*, an analysis of travel writing and Englishness, that "Africa [is] the mirror in which England must gaze at itself if it is to recover its essential values," (p. 186). See also Alison Blunt (1994), *Travel, Gender, and Imperialism: Mary Kingsley and West Africa*; Kristi Siegel (Ed.) (2002), *Issues in Travel Writing: Empire, Spectacle, and Displacement*; and James Duncan and Derek Gregory (Eds.) (2000), *Writes of Passage: Reading Travel Writing*.

8. My reading of this image is inspired by Wendy Kozol's argument in her 2003 conference paper to the American Studies Association Annual Meeting, "Anxiety and Comfort Under the Mushroom Cloud: Masculinity, Militarism, and National Belonging."

9. This ideological construction relies on a distinction between consumption and production, so that productive labor is not visible as value. It is ironic that it is precisely handwork that can also produce capitalist value for "authentic" crafts, especially in the context of travel. Obviously, this reading of class in the image is entirely ideological, as it in no way can imagine that the dancer's outfits might in fact be very expensive—or the President's suit a cheap product of the global assembly line.

10. In an image of the same event from a CBS News photo essay, the caption indicated that this event marked the playing of the "Star Spangled Banner" (see CBS News, 2003, image 7 of 20). The CBS News photo essay includes two images of this event. One (image 7 of 20) is a medium-range shot cropped to include only the presidents and their wives; the other (image 8 of 20) is a forced perspective through the space created by the saluting figure—Presidents Bush and Mbeki are in focus, while the rest of the frame is filled with the blurry shoulder and arm. This strategy even more forcefully situates the viewer as the saluting figure, but since Bush is more central to the image, draws an even stronger connection between the U.S. president and the salute.

11. This stop was the occasion for one of the most visible counternarratives to emerge from the trip. The disruptive effect of the security measures seemed to stand in ironic juxtaposition with the rhetoric of the Goree Island visit. For example, see Jonah Engle (2003).

12. Examples of coverage include B. Kemper (2003), "Bush Reaffirms AIDS Pledge in Botswana"; J. Donnelly (2003), "Bush Promises US Help in Africa's AIDS Battle"; B. Roth (2003), "Message Delivered"; and S. Thomma (2003), "Bush Vows Help on AIDS."

13. A full analysis of shifts in U.S. AIDS policy—and U.S. Africa policy—would need to detail the impact of evangelical Christian lobbying of the Bush administration.

14. The popularization of such policy rubrics in relation to HIV/AIDS also reflects the increasing predominance of national-security frames to address infectious disease. Ebola, SARS, and avian flu all reveal the impact of this model and its theoretical differences from the human-security frame promoted by human-rights approaches to health. For an example of policy analysis utilizing the concept of "failed states," see Stephen Krasner's and Carlos Pascual's (2005), "Addressing State Failure."

15. One possible connection that might be teased out is the relationship of the coverage of AIDS orphans in Africa and coverage of child-soldiers in Liberia and other armed conflicts. I do not mean to suggest that there are not real material issues facing children recruited into material organizations, but rather that the juxtaposition of representations of the strangely terrifying child-soldier and the AIDS orphan may produce a larger discourse about the "African child." What is potentially most insidious about the construction of African children within the framework of militarism is how little such narratives do to address the needs of those children. For an example of reporting on child soldiers, see Reuters' (2003) "Liberia's Child Soldiers Struggle to Rebuild Lives."

16. For an analysis of the trope of the reservoir, see M. Raimondo (1999).

17. "Not only have "millions of children...been orphaned," noted the *Atlanta Journal-Constitution*, but social unrest has the potential to turn adults into orphans, as in the case of a woman named "Daphne Moloi, who was infected by the only boyfriend she ever had...She felt, she said, like an orphan" (D. Melvin, 2003, p. A5). As geographer Karin Johnson (2002) noted, the emergence of AIDS in Africa as a national security issue in the late 1990s used "the quintessentially entwined US ideals of control and charity" to construct "military might as a form of virtue" (p. 90).

18. For more on this situation, see R. Cardelle et al. (2004), "Service-System Gaps for People With HIV/AIDS and Additional Health Challenges"; K. Heslin et al. (2004), "Racial and Ethnic Disparities in Access to Physicians With HIV-Related Expertise"; and L. Morales et al. (2004), "Sociodemographic Differences in Access to Care Among Hispanic Patients Who Are HIV Infected in the United States."

19. Susan Moeller (1999) developed the concept of compassion fatigue to describe media strategies that result in a desensitization and obfuscation of crisis. Her analysis is, in many ways, illuminating, and I do not mean to

dismiss the concept out of hand. I do, however, want to suggest that it may not be enough to assume that media imagery exhausts compassion, leading to the failure of advocacy. As Cindy Patton (1996) argued in *Fatal Advice*, compassion is a concept whose ideological work must be carefully evaluated in particular moments. It can be mobilized to support the status quo, as well as to challenge it.

Logistic Regression Analyses (Odds Ratios) for Likelihood of Having Seen Advertisement in Last 12 Months and Likelihood That Advertisement Prompted Physician Contact: Men and Women

Predictor	Seen/Heard Advertisement in Last 12 Months	Advertisement Prompted You to Speak to a Doctor
Sex (0 = M, 1 = F)	1.78*	1.29**
African American (0 = No, 1 = Yes)	0.47*	1.65**
Latino/Latina (0 = No, 1 = Yes)	0.32*	1.3
Education	1.94*	0.79**
Income	1.30*	1.0
Age	0.75**	0.73*
Health-insurance coverage (0 = No, 1 = Yes).	.971	0.82
Prescription-drug coverage (0 = No, 1 = Yes)	1.40	0.88
Take prescription drugs regularly (0 = No, 1 = Yes)	1.14	1.93***
Have regular doctor (0 = No, 1 = Yes)	1.05	1.17
Been diagnosed with chronic condition (0 = No, 1 = Yes)	1.56**	2.05*

(continued on next page)

(continued)

Predictor	Seen/Heard Advertisement in Last 12 Months	Advertisement Prompted You to Speak to a Doctor
Self-rated health (1 = Excellent, 2 = Very good, 3 = Good, 4 = Fair, 5 = Poor)	0.99	1.09
X^2	338.9	193.2
Pseudo R^2	.212	.112
N	2,605	2,291

*$p < .001$. **$p < .01$. ***$p < .05$.

Logistic Regression Analyses (Odds Ratios) for Likelihood of Having Seen Advertisement in Last 12 Months and Likelihood That Advertisement Prompted Physician Contact: Women Only

Predictor	Seen/Heard Advertisement in Last 12 Months	Advertisement Prompted You to Speak to a Doctor
African American (0 = No, 1 = Yes)	0.47**	2.15*
Latino/Latina (0 = No, 1 = Yes)	0.25*	1.44
Education	1.91**	0.77***
Income	1.47*	1.01
Age	0.66**	0.67*
Health-insurance coverage (0 = No, 1 = Yes)	0.69	1.45
Prescription-drug coverage (0 = No, 1 = Yes)	1.53	0.64
Take prescription drugs regularly (0 = No, 1 = Yes)	1.12	1.65*
Have regular doctor (0 = No, 1 = Yes)	1.48	0.91
Been diagnosed with chronic condition (0 = No, 1 = Yes)	2.11**	1.91*

(continued on next page)

(*continued*)

Predictor	Seen/Heard Advertisement in Last 12 Months	Advertisement Prompted You to Speak to a Doctor
Self-rated health (1 = Excellent, 2 = Very good, 3 = Good, 4 = Fair, 5 = Poor)	0.96	1.12
X^2	196.1	84.8
Pseudo R^2	.259	.093
N	1,329	1,193

$*p < .001.$ $**p < .01.$ $***p < .05.$

Logistic Regression Analyses (Odds Ratios)
for Likelihood That Physician Took Various Actions
as a Result of a DTCA-Induced Visit: Men and Women

Predictor	Doctor Prescribed Drug	Doctor Referred to a Specialist	Doctor Suggested Diet/ Exercise	Doctor Suggested Over-the- Counter Drug	Doctor Ordered Laboratory Test	Doctor Suggested Quitting Smoking/ Drinking
Sex (0 = M, 1 = F)	1.32	0.79	0.64**	0.84	0.74***	0.60**
African American (0 = No, 1 = Yes)	0.98	1.28	2.63*	0.87	1.13	1.22
Latino/Latina (0 = No, 1 = Yes)	1.13	1.66	2.49**	1.57	0.94	1.42
Education	1.04	1.08	1.22	0.82	1.19	0.71***
Income	1.01	0.91	0.94	0.97	0.93	0.90***
Age	0.81	1.08	1.23	0.81	1.88*	0.67**
Health-insurance coverage (0 = No, 1 = Yes)	1.06	1.01	0.47***	4.42**	0.78	1.08

(continued on next page)

(continued)

Predictor	Doctor Prescribed Drug	Doctor Referred to a Specialist	Doctor Suggested Diet/ Exercise	Doctor Suggested Over-the-Counter Drug	Doctor Ordered Laboratory Test	Doctor Suggested Quitting Smoking/ Drinking
Prescription-drug coverage (0 = No, 1 = Yes)	1.45	0.91	1.66	0.70	1.19	0.95
Take prescription drugs regularly (0 = No, 1 = Yes)	2.68*	1.30	0.95	0.62***	1.15	0.71
Have regular doctor (0 = No, 1 = Yes)	1.12	1.43	1.21	0.79	0.99	1.17
Been diagnosed with chronic condition (0 = No, 1 = Yes)	2.09*	1.70***	1.52*	0.63***	1.9**	2.21**
Self-rated health (1 = Excellent, 2 = Very good, 3 = Good, 4 = Fair, 5 = Poor)	1.00	1.54*	1.36*	0.93	1.36*	1.42*
X^2	79.4	86.9	78.8	38.9	108.9	89.8
Pseudo R^2	.129	.135	.118	.072	.161	.139
N	858	857	857	858	856	850

$*p < .001.$ $**p < .01.$ $***p < .05.$

Appendix D

Chronology of Governmental Actions on Trafficking

1994–1998: Authorities in Ukraine begin to take trafficking seriously after reports of multiple cases of illegal adoption of Ukrainian children.

March 24, 1998: Deputy Interior Minister M. Korniyenko initiates the creation of a special militia department on trafficking prevention. This is endorsed by the Ukrainian parliament in their vote to change the country's criminal code to include a definition of human trafficking and assign criminal responsibility to it (Article 124 1). As of 2001, this revised article reads as follows:

> Trafficking in persons and other illegal agreements regarding the transfer of a person means the sale, or otherwise paid transfer of a person, as well as any other illegal agreement concerning legal or illegal transport, with or without that person's consent, across the state border of Ukraine for further sale or transfer to another person or persons for the purpose of sexual exploitation, employment in the pornography business, engagement in criminal activity, indenture, adoption for commercial purposes, used in armed conflicts or labour exploitation.

April 13, 1998: The president of Ukraine, Leonid Kuchma, signs a law imposing criminal charges for the trafficking in human beings. It was previously adopted by the Ukrainian parliament on March 24 of that year.

June 15, 1999: Creation of the National Coordination Council on trafficking.

September 25, 1999: Ukrainian Cabinet of Ministers launches a complex program on women and children trafficking prevention named the Comprehensive Program to Prevent Trafficking in Women and Children.

December 2000: Ukraine signs the United Nations Convention against Transnational Organized Crime, and its accompanying Protocol to Prevent, Suppress and Punish Trafficking in Persons, Especially Women and Children.

February 20, 2001: The president and the Parliament of Ukraine express support for the idea of amending the Criminal Code of Ukraine. According to the proposed changes, a new type of criminal activity was to be introduced, relating to the organization of illegal trafficking of foreign citizens from Ukraine.

September 1, 2001: The amendment of Article 149 of the Criminal Code suggests punishing people guilty of trafficking with 2–5 years of prison or a fine.

2002–2003: The Interior Ministry of Ukraine takes part in Eastern and Western European international operation "Sunflower," organized by Europol in an effort to close the channels of women trafficked from Ukraine to Italy to further sexual exploitation. Also, the ministry participates in "Mirazh," "Mirazh–2003," and "Mirazh–2004," all organized by the Southeast European Cooperative Initiative (SECI) Center in order to prevent and fight human trafficking and illegal migration on the territory of Southern-Eastern Europe.

June 5, 2002: Cabinet of Ministers approves the Complex Anti-Trafficking Programme for 2002–2005. Its main aims are to improve prevention of trafficking, support victims, and facilitate police work on the investigation of trafficking crimes. It includes an explicit role for NGOs and international organizations in implementing various aspects of the program.

December 2002: A general antitrafficking cooperation program for 2003–2005 is signed by the International Labour Organization (ILO) and the Interior Ministry of Ukraine.

December 25, 2002: Establishment of Inter-Agency Coordinating Council for the Prevention of Trafficking in Persons, a permanent advisory body under the Cabinet of Ministers of Ukraine. Its head is the Minister of Family, Children, and Youth Affairs.

October 21–22, 2002: International conference called *Preventing Human Trafficking—Economic Problems and the Ways of Their Solution* is organized by USAID, the Academy of Education Development, the government of Ukraine, and, in particular, the State Committee on Family and Youth in Ukraine, along with La Strada.

June 27, 2003: Cabinet Resolution on "Establishing Standard Rules for a Rehabilitation Centre for Trafficked Persons."

February 4, 2004: Ukraine ratifies the UN Protocol to Prevent, Suppress and Punish Trafficking in Persons, especially Women and Children, deemed the Palermo Protocol.

November 17, 2004: Cabinet of Ministers Decree (No. 1559 3045) "On rights and interests of citizens that go abroad for work, and on adoptions by foreigners children for the period until 2005."

December 2004: The Ukrainian government establishes an advisory antitrafficking working group to improve coordination of the largely ineffectual Inter-Ministerial Group.

October 24, 2005: Family, Youth & Sports Minister Yurii Pavlenko reports to the Interagency Coordinating Committee for combating human trafficking. A comprehensive antitrafficking program for 2006–2011 is launched. A special telephone hotline is established to advise those who will travel abroad.

2005: The Parliament of Ukraine discusses the Concept of the National Target-Specific Program to Counter Trade in Humans in 2006–2010 and discusses a plan to set up the National Coordinator Bureau for combating human trafficking.

April 10, 2006: Ministry of Internal Affairs Trafficking Crimes Department launches a telephone hotline.

March 7, 2007: The government adopts a National Anti-Trafficking in Persons Program for the period until 2010.

March 17, 2007: The parliamentary committee of law enforcement holds a roundtable called "Problems with Ratification of the Council of Europe Convention on Anti-Trafficking."

February 27, 2008: The parliamentary committee of law enforcement holds a roundtable called "Implementation of the State Policy of Anti-Trafficking in Persons: State, Problems, Perspectives."

LIST OF CONTRIBUTORS

COEDITORS BIOGRAPHY

Cindy Patton holds the Canada Research Chair in Community Culture and Health at Simon Fraser University in British Columbia, where she is a professor of sociology & anthropology and women's studies. She is also the senior scholar of the Michael Smith Foundation for Health research. Dr. Patton was an AIDS activist and community organizer throughout the 1980s, and subsequently worked as a researcher and scholar. Her publications include: *Inventing AIDS* (1990); *Last Served? Gendering the HIV Pandemic* (1994); *Fatal Advice* (1996); *Queer Diasporas* (with Benigno Sanchez-Eppler, 2000); *Globalizing AIDS* (2002) and *Cinematic Identity* (2007). She is currently the head of the Health Research and Methods Training Facility, a qualitative research lab with a focus on community-based research.

Helen Loshny is a PhD candidate in the Department of Women's Studies at Simon Fraser University, where she researches in the Health Research and Methods Training Facility. Her areas of interest include women's reproductive health and critical perspectives on clinical practice. She is currently coediting the volume *Clinical Spaces and Agents* with C. Patton. An article coauthored with C. Patton (currently in press) will shortly appear in the *Canadian Journal of Nursing Research*.

CONTRIBUTORS' BIOGRAPHIES

Rachel Askew is a PhD candidate in Sociology at Emory University in Atlanta. She has recently coauthored "Latinas at Work: Issues of Gender, Ethnicity and Class" with I. Browne, for the volume *Gender, Ethnicity and Race in the Workplace* (M. Karsten (Ed.), 2006).

Irene Browne is an associate professor of sociology at Emory University. She is the editor of the volume *"Latinas and African American Women at Work: Race, Gender, and Economic Inequality* (1999), which was selected as an outstanding academic book of 1999 by Choice magazine. She has authored various chapters in edited volumes, such as "Labor Market Inequality: Intersections of Gender, Race and Class" (coauthored with J. Misra) in *Blackwell Companion to*

Inequalities (M. Romero & E. Margolis (Eds.), 2005), and her articles have also appeared in journals such as the *Annual Review of Sociology* (2003) and *Social Science Research* (2001).

Lisa Diedrich is an assistant professor of women's studies at Stony Brook University. She is the author of *Treatments: Language, Politics, and the Culture of Illness* (2007) and is currently completing *Feminist Time Against Nation Time,* a volume she coedited with Victoria Hesford. Lisa's writing has also appeared in academic journals including *Literature and Medicine* (2001, 2004). Her current research investigates how breast cancer on Long Island emerged historically through complex practices, including medical, political, scientific, economic, and affective practices.

Diane Goldstein is a professor of folklore at Memorial University of Newfoundland and is cross-appointed to Memorial University's School of Medicine. She is author of *Once Upon A Virus: AIDS Legends and Vernacular Risk Perception* (2004), coeditor (with Cindy Patton and Heather Worth) of a special issue of *Sexuality Research and Social Policy* entitled "Reckless Vectors: The Infecting Other in HIV/AIDS Law" (2005), and editor of one of the earliest interdisciplinary anthologies on HIV/AIDS, entitled *Talking AIDS: Interdisciplinary Perspectives on Acquired Immune Deficiency Syndrome* (1991). Diane has been extensively involved in HIV/AIDS priority-setting and policy-making initiatives over the last 20 years including a 3-year appointment to the Canadian National Planning and Priorities Forum for HIV/AIDS.

Olena Hankivsky is an associate professor of political science at Simon Fraser University, where she also serves as the Director of the Institute for Critical Studies in Gender and Health. Her work examines the practical implications of a care ethic for a range of policy issues, both in Canada and in the larger, global framework. She is the author of *Social Policy and the Ethic of Care* (2004) and coauthor of *The Dome of Silence: Sexual Harassment and Abuse in Sport* (2000). Her work has also appeared in numerous academic journals, including the *Canadian Journal of Political Science* (2005) and the *Journal of Nursing Law* (2002).

Marina Morrow is an assistant professor in the Faculty of Health Sciences at Simon Fraser University. Her specialization is in mental health with foci on women, access to health services, critical health policy, and health reform. Dr. Morrow's articles have appeared in a range of journals including *The Journal of Critical Social Policy* and *Women's Health International.* She coedited the book *Women's Health in Canada: Critical Perspectives on Theory and Policy* (2007) with O. Hankivsky and C. Varcoe.

Meredith Raimondo is an assistant professor of the Comparative American Studies Program at Oberlin College. Her work has appeared in *Environment and Planning D* and *Gender, Place and Culture* as well as anthologies such as *Just Advocacy: Women's Human Rights, Transnational Feminisms*, the *Politics of Representation* and *Carryin' On in the Lesbian and Gay South*. She is currently working on a book about the U.S. media's representation of the geography of HIV/AIDS.

Heather Worth is the Deputy Director of the National Centre for HIV in Social Research of Australia. Her research is primarily in the areas of HIV, gender, and sexuality, with a recent emphasis on HIV and global politics. She is the author of *Gay Men, Sex and HIV in New Zealand* (2003) and has coedited a number of edited volumes, including *Baudrillard west of the dateline* (2002) with V. Grace and L. Simmons; *From Z to A: Zizek and the Antipodes* (2005) with L. Simmons and M. Mollow; and "Reckless Vectors: Aids and Criminality" (2005), a special issue of the *Journal of Sexuality Research and Social Policy*, with C. Patton and D. Goldstein. Her work has also appeared regularly in many prominent scholarly journals, including *AIDS Prevention and Education* (2003), the *Journal of Bisexuality* (2002), and the *Journal of Sociology* (2002).

INDEX

patients (*continued*)
    psychiatric, 16–17, 151. *See also*
      psychiatry
    relationship with doctors, 31, 59,
      95–98, 106. *See also* doctors;
      relationship with patients
pharmaceutical companies. *See* drug
    companies
pharmaceutical industry, 35
    advertising. *See* DTCA
Philadelphia (film), 225–226
post-structuralism, 6–7, 9, 148, 158
post-traumatic stress disorder,
    155–157, 162, 172, 190
poverty, 3–4, 20, 122, 126, 186–187,
    236, 244
    and women, 15, 19, 186–187
power, 11–12, 21, 148, 163,
    177, 243
    distribution, 10
    and gender. *See* gender; and
      power
Powers, Richard, 13, 88–91, 93, 97,
    100, 102–109, 114n1, 115nn8–9
    turn from science to literature,
      89–91
practices of witnessing. *See*
    witnessing; practices of
prescription drugs, 51, 53–55, 66, 76
    adherence. *See* HIV; drug
      regimens
    cost, 55–56
    demand, 55
    marketing changes, 53, 76
    side effects, 56
privatization, 4, 103, 179. *See also*
    neoliberalism
product warnings, 11, 26, 39–44
protease inhibitors, 118, 126

psychiatry, 16, 148–149, 154–155,
    158, 161, 171n1, 172n8
    diagnostic categories, 154–157,
      159, 162, 171n2, 172n11
    stigma associated with, 157, 162,
      171n1
    discourse, 147–148, 152, 158–159
    feminist critiques, 147–148, 151,
      153–154, 156–157, 160–161,
      171n2
    feminist changes to, 151–153,
      155, 158, 161, 163
    institutions, 16–17, 151, 158–159
    psychiatrists, 150–151, 159,
      171n1
    survivor movement, 147–148,
      152, 157, 163, 171n1. *See
      also* activism; anti-psychiatry
      movement
    treatments within, 152, 157,
      159–160
psychology, 149, 151, 152, 154, 159

race, 2, 12, 52, 57, 120, 136–137,
    162, 223, 225–232,
    236–237, 241
racism, 2, 237, 253n7
    scientific, 2
randomized trials. *See* clinical trials
research, 9
    centers for, 2
    practices, 7, 108
    results, 9
Roy, Arundhati, 89, 114n4

science, 2, 6, 89–90, 107, 110, 139
    alternative, 3, 26, 102
    translation of, 3, 9
    and society, 9

Printed in the United States
211538BV00002B/4/P

9 781934 844038